...and N(
Cannot Laugh
Anymore

by

Mark Griffith

Cover art by Rod Horne
Cover design by Charli Vince
www.charlivince.com

Dedication

For my son, Noel George Frederick.

Have fun and enjoy your life, son,
I will be with you wherever you are.

Contents

Introduction by Sheila Griffith

Our son, Mark returned to England in 2008 after working overseas for several years. None of us knew then just how fortunate that was to be.

He came to live with us in Norwich and found work locally, eventually saving enough to buy a flat in the City centre.

He married a young lady he had met whilst working in Albania and in August 2010 they celebrated the birth of their son Noel.

Mark then bought a house with a garden for his child, which they moved into in April 2012.

It was later that year that Mark fell ill with a sore throat and bad cough.

After x-rays and a scan it was discovered he had throat cancer.

He was given this news on December 24th 2012.

Mark started to think about his life and decided to write his story.

My 46 and a half years of struggle against bad luck,
misfortune and wives

by

Mark Griffith

Actually, given that there will be some of you who read this with a smidgen of historical knowledge you will have realised just who and which book I have badly paraphrased.

Given that I wish to avoid another court case then let's just call this book:

…and Now I Just Cannot Laugh Anymore

by

Mark Griffith

Introduction:

The bit you look through quickly to see if the rest is worth reading and, if not, at least, you can pretend you have.

It happens every time you have some bad luck. It could be ill health, personal grief or a job re-organisation at Norfolk County Council,[1] it doesn't matter. There is always a moronic friend or family member who says to you: "Look on the bright side there is always someone else worse off than you." That someone is, in fact, me.

This book will detail in simple, factual terms, and with self-deprecating humour, what a waste of space I am – or just how unlucky I have been. You get to pick in the end! It is not an autobiography. I am not famous; at least, I have avoided that humiliation. I am also not quite dead and, knowing my luck; there will be yet more disasters before I get to die. Then I will find out that there is an afterlife, and it takes place in a bar permanently stuck at closing time and filled with dumb, arrogant people all wanting money or telling me how wonderful they are.

This book will not follow a strict pattern of going through my life; from early days to school, to my first

---

[1] Organisation responsible for Local Government in the county of Norfolk in the United Kingdom. Administrative centre: Norwich, pop. 213,166 at the 2011 Census.

job and so on. We'll hit just the highlights to prove the above point: that I am the "worse off" person that I mentioned. It's a tale told with humour because you are supposed to laugh at me. I have long since realised that you do not laugh with a person. No, you take the piss out of them. You now have the opportunity to luxuriate in taking the mickey out of me.

Please do not look for any message of hope or a cure or bravery in this. My reaction to the whole of life is pretty much the same - humorous. It's just the way that I am. However, if, through these ramblings of a madman, some of you do get a good laugh, then that is a positive gain. God forbid, but some of you may face similar circumstances to mine, or have a loved one in the same position. If that's the case, and a couple of funny lines out of this somewhere helps you, or the general idiotic attitude is of assistance, then that's great. We will all face this "end of life" scenario sometime. So, no counselling and no big hugs: I am English. I do not cry and I shake hands. If the god of cock-ups had wanted me to be a wailing waste of space at this moment, he would have made me Italian or Albanian. And if he wanted me to talk utter bullshit, and tell you that I have the answer to everything then he would have made me American.

Now you can chuck this in the bin. On the other hand, if you want to read some funny dirt about me, then dive right in. I've included some ridiculous non-smutty material as well, so the planners and legal people I know have something to read. Remember this is factual, not fictional. All that follows really happened to me. This book was very easy to write. All I have done is to recall some of the funnier incidents and write them down. That's it. My life has seriously been this stupid. Please enjoy. Shall we begin?

Chapter One: The Start of It All

In the beginning, the Lord Great Almighty created the Universe. (Just trust me with this and where it is going). He saweth the Universe that he had created and saweth that it was goodly with all the stars and moons. But it was an empty place so He decided to create a planet. Above this, He created the Heavens and filled them with all manner of wonderful birds and they were all happy. But He thought it needed something more so he created the seas and filled them with all manner of fish. Like the birds, they were of all colours and much beauty and they were all happy. But still as He looked down He thought the planet needed yet more. So He created the continents and filled them with all manner of wonderful, magnificent plants and animals to roam and grow and fill the place with great beauty. Of the beasts He had created He made one even greater than all the others and called it Man. Now as He looked down all was perfect.

Exactly. All was perfect. Just damn perfect. As the little robin red breast passed the great golden eagle and asked, "How are you?" then the answer had to be "I am wonderful". As the whale passed the goldfish and asked, "How are you?" then the answer remained "perfect". And in like manner, Prince Charles[2] passed the tree and asked, "How are you?" The tree did not answer because

---

[2] Prince of Wales and heir to the throne of the United Kingdom.

it was a tree and this particular Prince may be a little mad. But God got the point. All was perfect. No being had anything to compare their happiness with, or contrast it against, and that was not perfect. So the Almighty thought to Himself: What can I do about this?

The answer: create a subspecies for all creatures that is worse off than the others so the beautiful ones can always feel better about themselves. For example; Prince Charles got a brother called Andrew[3], the fish got plankton, and the birds got wasps. All of these subspecies sit at the bottom of the pile. They get to make everyone else feel good about their situation. It is their role in life.

For the greatest of all his creatures, Man, he created the species we know as 'Unlucky Bastard', a sort of local government employee of the world. Throughout the ages, there have always been 'Unlucky Bastards.' They are always in the wrong place at the wrong time. There was the man who was in the Hiroshima district when the first atomic bomb went off, and then went to Nagasaki to recover! The man who is always struck by lightning, no matter where he goes to be safe. These 'Unlucky Bastards' suffer great misery.

Then in 1966, the Almighty realised that the world was indeed going down the pan of the universal toilet. He

---

[3] Prince Andrew, younger brother of Charles.

needed a 'Uber Unlucky Bastard' to cover the full range of cock-ups. Then all his favoured creations would not feel so bad about the disasters that were befalling them in ever increasing numbers.

On April 23rd 1966, the world darkened just a smidge, and the wolves howled just a little with worried concern. With a squeak and a scream, I was born: 'Uber Disaster Man'.

Chapter Two: Birth and Early Childhood

As I said, this is no autobiography. But one does have to start at some point in the league of disasters so we might as well start with my birth. A comedian once said that the way to be a good stand up is to take a little truth from your life and just expand upon that. There is no expansion involved here; all of this is actually true. I agree, none of this makes me a comedian, however, it does make this book very easy to write!

So; my birth in April 1966. My mother had had three previous miscarriages. For some reason, I have it in my head that they were all boys. But the important point here is that if this were happening in the 21st Century, then we'd be looking at a woman and an unborn child surrounded by a serious medical team in a dedicated hospital with many machines making silly noises and drawing pretty pictures. Instead, we had a little cottage hospital[4] that my Dad served as vicar. Despite his wife's previous medical history they told him on the great day of reckoning to clear off and come back tomorrow. So he decided to go skating with some blonde bird[5] instead. That was his story, anyway!

---

[4] Typically, a small medical establishment serving a rural area of the United Kingdom.

[5] Collaquilism for 'Woman' much favoured in the UK in the 1960s and 1970s.

Given the hospital was straight out of Camberwick Green[6], the only assistance likely to be generally available is your own GP[7] strolling onto the ward, smoking his pipe. Well, guess what? Even the doctor had decided that a holiday was preferable to my birth. But it's still a hospital, right? Albeit in Toytown. So surely some help must be available given the dire medical history of the patient? No dear, no. First bite out of my good fortune cookie is a flu virus that has left just one member of staff available.

The second chunk out of that ever-decreasing cookie is that the substitute doctor is convinced that I am so keen to remain in the comfort of my mother that nothing will happen for another 24 hours. However, the problem with that diagnosis was that my mother was a professional ballerina and was used to pain. She is also very middle-class English and, therefore, did not want to complain too much. These days, the most miserable, lowest form of life that spawns its offspring will scream the place down for no apparent reason other than they saw it happen on Oprah. But no, my mother, who had a reason to do so, decides to be polite. So we are now down to two people involved in a potentially complex medical situa-

---

[6] A 1966 UK children's television programme featuring stop-motion puppets. Not known for their expertise in medical matters.

[7] General Medical Practicioner.

tion. My Mum and a nurse, and a whole history of disastrous births.

Time to move up the cavalry: Dad. The family story goes that, as my father was skating with his blonde partner on the ice rink, he got a premonition that there was a problem. Now this is great, and it may be what happened. Lights from the heavens of the Bristol ice rink may have shone down on him like they did on Saul on the road to Damascus (or Brian on the way to Kingswood if you will). But, as I am a genetic imprint of my Dad, I can't help but consider some other possibilities: 1. 'The pub has shut, and I am going to have to leave.' 2. 'The blonde has just told me to clear off, and I'm going to have to leave.' 3. 'The blonde's boyfriend has turned up, and this will just turn nasty, so I m going to have to leave.' Whatever the reason, the vicar of the little cottage hospital turned up on time.

So, despite the medical history which indicated major catastrophe, I was born with the able assistance of my mother, a nurse found wandering around a bit, and an errant father. I screamed a lot, and everyone was happy. It was the end of my luck.

As a matter of interest, my birth resulted in the complete destruction of my mother internally. I seemed to have this effect on women! That, and the ability to send them mad. While Mum lost various organs, I carried on oblivious. She had to have operations. These went wrong and almost killed her. What a wonderful son! So, at the grand old age of her early 30s, my mother was minus a womb and various other bits and pieces. Unfortunately, the medical profession missed out one part of the repair process: hormones. Ladies, I ask you for just a moment to imagine what that must have been like for her. Gentlemen, please imagine what it was like for my Dad!! But all was sorted in the end. I did not actually destroy their marriage with my birth, just enhanced some major areas of future negotiation between them. Poor buggers. The fact that my father did not strangle me during the opening five years of my life is a wondrous thing.

To complete this section on my birth, I should highlight another point. As I mentioned before, the Almighty has created me as the 'Uber Disaster Man', or in English: the ultimate cock up. Of course, you will require some proof of this. Otherwise, you may read the rest of this book and think I am just a man who has had a couple of accidents and is so boring that he sits at home and writes about it. (Hang on, I am at home alone doing exactly that; must get back to the pub!) But let me finish the birth bit before I do.

My mother suffers from asthma, and this means regular check-ups. After all her medical misadventures, she was chatting with her doctor during one of these sessions. After reading her file and all her test results, he said:

"Well you are doing OK at the moment, but I am so sorry that you could never have children." The wolves howled once more! Medically, my mother could never have had a child, and yet I exist!

So now I want my money back. The three wise men never turned up at the hospital, and the presents were shit. Providing me with an excess of shepherds and sheep is no excuse. We lived next door to Wales, so they were going to turn up anyway. Also, my carpentry skills are bollocks. Ok, I accept I do have the ability to turn wine into far more wine. Also, I married a Jew, which I suppose, brings me a little bit closer to being a member of the religion. And I acknowledge that I have been crucified many times by various solicitors and wives, and have risen again, so I give you that bit as well.

Or we could consider it this way. My father was a vicar, his brother was too, and his youngest brother was a lay preacher. That's not looking good, is it? The movie ends with a shot of me just born into the hand of my father. He's dressed in full ministerial robes and surrounded by 30 colleagues in hooded cloaks outside Bristol University Chapel. They are chanting. Just call me Damien for short.

But let's say it was the Almighty who foisted me on to this planet with the means at His disposal. I am sure that my relationship to the deity is somewhat dubious, though; perhaps I am the runt of the family? But I had arrived. So was it was time to prove my worth as the subspecies of 'Unlucky Bastard.'? Not quite yet.

For most people, not a lot happens in their childhood of long-term significance, and it seemed to be the same for me. I had a great time. I had a sister who, as a baby, bore a distinct resemblance to Winston Churchill. I spent hours farting in her face and locking her in her room. Unfortunately, she quickly grew up and beat the shit out of me. She is now a little less than 6'2". And I am a massive 5'7".

In all honesty, my childhood was great. No complaints. School was fine. I got on with most people and enjoyed the company of a wide range of kids, which was what I was taught to do. I liked everyone. All this took place in the early 1970s in a small town called Kettering. I did the lot; from attempting to chat up girls to making a complete idiot of myself. I stored up a treasury of embarrassing moments that I could cringe at later in life. As we all do. But the Almighty decided that I was slacking. It was time for me to be of assistance to the world.

All boys ride go-carts. I did it at 20 miles an hour down a side road with my head bouncing on the tarmac. Most kids would have broken an arm or a leg or whatever. No, not me. I survive intact. Nothing wrong with me. At least not for some weeks. Then all hell breaks loose. I wake up suddenly in the middle of the night. I crawl to my parent's room, dribbling uncontrollably and eating carpet. After my collapse, I fling myself all over the place. There is significant vomiting and urination.

Welcome to epilepsy. I had managed to damage my brain. Permanently. Total joy! A future of drugs being stuffed into me to calm my brain down. As you will gather by the end of the book, these may not have been a total success, but just imagine if I'd forgotten to take them. I'm not sure if this was connected to my eyesight issues but around the same time, I had to start wearing the famous thick, black prescription NHS[8] glasses with a sticking plaster added to hold the broken frames together.

Now I was going to school looking like a major clown, and with the full possibility of collapsing like one. Super, God, and thanks for the ego boost. But this is just minor rubbish really, and, of course, I overcame it and adapted in a short period. I became the immediate and most obvious butt of everyone's jokes. Yes, the Great One had assigned me to save the School Wallys[9] from such a fate, and I was so happy to perform the task. I had always felt that I was different from other kids anyway. I was so full of confidence that I could talk my way

---

[8] The National Health Service: the UK's world famous free medical service; currently targetted by businessmen and politicians determined to make lots of money from other people's misfortunes.

[9] Derogatory term for kids at school who aren't any good at sport.

out of any tricky situation. On the other hand, perhaps these were the circumstances which forced me to learn how to waffle for Queen and Country.

For most people, this sort of setback is the first, and perhaps last, hiccup they will have to deal with in their lifetime. They would be rather sad about it, apparently. So I have been told. Even complain that they had been hard done by. Wasters.

Right. Let's rock on to another subject. How about...

Chapter Three: Transport

To be entirely honest this section is not so much about bad luck as bad timing. Some weird things have happened to me relating to travel, but they could have happened to anyone. It's just very unlikely that other people would end up in quite the same situation as me. To give you an example; I once drove a tube train on London's Northern Line. I'm not qualified to do it; it was a mate of mine who was the driver. One day he stopped his train at Clapham South station and saw me on the platform. He offered me a seat in the cab. I ended up driving the train to the station where I wanted to go. Imagine doing that now!

Another time a different friend and I were in the middle of the Sudan with a jeep that decided it was not going to work. All our manly remarks about the thingy connection requiring some more fiddly do dah[10] were in vain. Our prayers to every god known to man seemed to be equally effective. But, eventually, it decided to move. If it hadn't our last memories of this world would have been of the famous mini black pyramids. And there are other silly examples. But these are not the stories you want to hear from the muck up king!

---

[10] A technical term.

There are three transport catastrophes that spring to mind and a fourth if you count my lost week with two Danish girls on a train. I lost them, and they ended up in my bed in Norwich while I was in Norway!! We can re-visit that in another section. Unfortunately, these things always result in an emotional breakdown for me.

Driving a Car - My Way

I never enjoyed driving that much, but I learnt at the age of 17. The epilepsy held off and allowed me to do so. I believe I was allowed this foray into the world of mo-torised transport just to ensure a level of humiliation significant enough that it would always allow others to think, "Well, at least, I wasn't as stupid as Mark". This outcome is a general principle of life that I should never forget.

My memory of the first occasion is a little hazy, but I believe it was a friends 17th or 18th birthday party, which was being held in the Dereham[11] area. The only way to get there was to drive, and it was my job to do it. As I recall, 30 years ago there wasn't much of an issue with mad kids driving. Until that particular night.

---

[11] A small market town 15 miles west of the city of Norwich.

The invitation for the party read "smart dress". So I wore one of my sister's dresses. The guy next to me in the front wore his father's ministerial robes (his father being a vicar at Her Majesty's Prison in Norwich). The lad sat behind me was a good-looking Turkish bloke wearing a swimming costume, complete with snorkel and flippers. We also picked up a beautiful blonde girl in all her finery, who was immediately worried about the sanity of her choice of a lift to the party. Strange, that.

I drove to the ring road that leads out of Norwich with the window wound down looking as cool as one can in a royal blue dress. I was prepared for an evening of great fun and joviality. Then we came to a thing called a roundabout. My brain checked out immediately. I rammed my foot down, believing we could fit into a small space between the oncoming traffic. We hit gravel, and the world went slow. The car spun. I saw a priest ducking for cover behind my dashboard and a swimmer in my back mirror sticking a snorkel in his ear.

The car had somehow managed to miss all the other ve-hicles. There was a moment of silence. We were sat on the other side of the roundabout facing the wrong way into the traffic. But we were all still alive, and there was no significant smell of excrement in the car. All is OK. No, not quite. Out ran Mr. "I spend my life looking out of my window" man to see what had happened, and to justify his pathetic little existence. He stuck his head in the driver's side window and saw a transvestite, a vicar, a semi-naked bloke with a flipper in his mouth and a gorgeous hostess. I blew him a kiss and attempted to pull away. We weren't in Hollywood of course, so I accomplished our escape only after a two hundred-point turn. No one would drive back with me that night. Apart from the vicar. He reckoned it was better than being pissed so he would try it again. I didn't do much more driving after that!

Another Car Journey

I am not really sure that this story doesn't belong in the sexual disasters section, but the transport category is a little weak in comparison. The only other appropriate memory involving a car is seeing my sister drive off and leave my father and me in a blizzard outside Thursford. So, to bolster this part of the book, I include it here as yet another example of the scenario of the 'Unlucky Bastard' and transport.

Three friends and I had been to a party in Norwich. Again, I was somewhere around 18 years of age. Luck was with us that night it seemed. Three very attractive girls had latched onto us. By 'attractive', I mean we were well out of our league. They did not have two heads, and there was no obvious webbing between their fingers. They had arms and legs in the correct places.

Their faces were without scars, and there was no sign of the bubonic plague. They were also speaking independently and did not have carers with them. Somehow, they'd been convinced to get into my friend's car and head to the beach, some 10 miles away, for rumpty tumpty.[12]

Naturally the fine lady I was with was the best looking of the lot! Both of her. Yes, we'd all had a couple of plastic bottles of Strongbow[13] and had stumbled across a massive tin of lager. I assumed the driver was fine. By that I mean I didn't give a hoot how drunk he was, provided he could get his car to the beach where I might get my vile horny little way.

Again, this was 30 years ago, and I presumed everything was fine. Circumstances never seem to change, only my point of view. Now, of course, I assume that everything is not fine and work backwards from there. But, back then, my little head was telling me that the driver was a Methodist, who had passed the police's advanced driving test. Oh, No. Big Oh No. Seriously not the case at all.

_____

[12] A Norfolk collaquilism that means exactly what you think it does.

[13] A British cider. The author is likely referring to the 2 litre bottle.

We headed into the countryside with some heavy metal band playing on the cassette deck. Then we had to turn a corner. Up until that corner, I had a warm feeling of good beer drunk, good music, fine conversation, the sweet lips of an attractive girl and the prospect of major sex. After that corner, I was faced with 3 screaming girls, a driver in shock and another mate wandering up the road at 2 a.m who is about to announce to the residents of a nearby village that he's going to kill himself.

I assumed something at that point but asked the question anyway. Yes, sex was out of the question. Having resolved that immediate issue, I ensured there were no real casualties. The girls quickly decided that the driver actually wanted to kill them, so I left that debate to continue and did a quick reconnaissance of the scene. We had hit a garden wall and totalled it. Now, in the real world, you simply calm all the people down and mention the matter to the owners of the wall in question. However, in the world of the insane, you drag the car off the wall, hit the driver until he starts communicating again, and hurl the girls back into the car. It was not my finest plan. Garden walls are not made of Lego, and it was obvious that it had been well fucked up. Similarly, the car would now only turn left. Ok, so not a disaster, I thought. If we keep left, we can get back to my mates' house, and stay there. I can still get rumpty tumpty. We can resolve all other issues in the morning. The idiot in my underpants was doing all my thinking for me.

We did get to my friend's house. What he had forgotten to mention was that his mother wished to kill him. Literally kill him. She had a shotgun in her arms. So, there we were. A driver who could not speak, just dribble; three crying girls claiming all forms of hell were coming down on them and a teenage boy in the midst of some macabre death dance with his mother. A contest she was most definitely going to win. Fortunately, the mother and I had met before, and I calmed her down. My success was probably based on the fact that I was the only one who was not screaming or dribbling. And the one thing I do have; the winning smile that mothers like. I explained the situation with a quiver of hope, not of saving the others' lives you understand, but of my own personal sexual gratification. Hope of this liaison was wilting, but I was holding on. The mother agreed we could stay if I removed her son immediately the next morning. Of course, the girls went to another room. And, of course, my dream of sexual conquest died a horrible and pathetic death. But the fun and games weren't over yet.

I was stuck with dribbling driver and the mental case mate whose mum hates him. Punishment, enough? Of course not. We might have forgotten about what had happened to the wall, but others were not so absent-minded. Like the avengers of doom, the Norfolk Constabulary descended upon us. Please try to imagine attempting to explain to a policeman why you drove a car that only turned left away from a crime scene. Try to explain why local witnesses were claiming they had heard death threats being shouted by the roughly dressed youths involved. I looked at the driver, said it was all his fault and went to bed!

But this didn't work. The police had latched onto me as the only member of the group that was capable of speech and did not belong in an asylum. Therefore, I can still recall a long and deranged conversation with them as I tried to explain the evening's events. The police became more concerned about my friend's mother. She had reappeared by then, and assuming that everything was her son's fault, once again commenced to threaten him with all forms of hell. I do not recall the shotgun making a repeat appearance, thank the gods. I think I phoned my Mum, got home sometime later that morning, and proceeded to hide from the world.

It's certainly the biggest loss of a potentially good night due to a car accident that I have ever experienced. And without a doubt, the most confused mess arising from one. If ever a teenage boy feels hard done by when a guaranteed evening of sexual activity goes wrong, then please refer him to this story. It's always a worse case scenario when 'Uber Disaster Man' is involved.

Epileptic Fit on a Plane

There are a limited number of examples of bad luck from my life that involve transport. Most of those that I have experienced could have happened to other people. No doubt the two I have already mentioned are common enough to most blokes of my age; with variations of course. This one is slightly different and was a major personal embarrassment.

I used to travel a lot on planes. I bloody hate airports, but flying is fine. When I worked for the Foreign Office, I did need to travel that way, if only to get home. One trip from Bulgaria to London via Vienna went badly wrong.

Boarding the plane, I experienced no problems. I sat down and got the peanuts out. The plane took off. Everything was normal. Then I drifted off to sleep. Unfortunately, epilepsy usually strikes me when I'm in the process of waking up. On this occasion, my return to reality was accompanied by the realisation that a fit was on its way. And this was not going to be a little episode that I could cover up, but a major blockbuster. And I am on a plane.

I got up from my seat like a drunken walrus and spluttered a few words to a stewardess. She was already aiming herself at me as I dribbled and started to fall. Somehow, I ended up near the cockpit listening to a discussion containing the phrase: "Should we return?" At last, I managed to get out some words. "No, it's just a fit; keep going". Well, you might think that was the end of it. Any epileptics reading this will know that usually everything is fine a few minutes after a seizure. Apart from about 150 people on a plane thinking that you are demented. Finally, I was dragged back to my seat. The plane flew on.

Welcome to Air Austria. At Vienna airport, the plane was held, and an ambulance arrived. Then the bloody medics wheeled me off in a wheelchair thing. I was pushed through the busy airport to the medical centre, where I was subjected to a battery of tests. Now, I am used to having medical things poked into me, but I only had an hour and a half between flights, and they wanted to check the lot. Thank God, I hadn't had a beer or slept with a goat that day. Finally, I was wheeled out and dropped in the centre of the terminal. I wasn't allowed to walk before, but now I was removed from the chair in front of thousands of people. Of course, I walked fine. Arise Lazarus! I looked like a total pillock.[14]

I have learnt a big thing from this. I try to avoid long journeys on public transport without a member of my own family. God bless my Mummy. She has hidden

---

[14] Derogatory Bristish term for idiot. Believed to have been adopted in the 16th Century and derived from the Norwegian 'pillcock'.

these fits of mine from a number of coach drivers on trips to London before and since. We just carry on, avoiding all the paperwork, the enforced stops for health and safety and the no doubt hideous insurance issues. But a big warning to everyone else; never travel with me.

Transport is a nightmare if you travel with the risk of the kind of public embarrassment that follows me. But should you trip over in the train station, or feel sick on the coach, then please remember the 'Uber Disaster Man'. I am the man who is worse off than you.

Chapter Four: Employment

What to talk about next? Given that the majority of you reading this will be my work colleagues, I think it is time for you to have a laugh at my employment history. We will, therefore, cast away my Curriculum Vitae, and any possibility of a career within County Hall.[15] These are the highlights of the mistakes, bad fortune and complete humiliation of my career as Mark 'Unlucky Bastard' Griffith, the "worker".

As with almost all of us, I started work at 16. I was employed at Greens electrical store in Debenhams[16] for a couple of years while at Sixth Form[17]. I had great fun. It was a shame that I knew nothing about Hifi, TVs or videos. I did know that the Sinclair 48K RAM computer was rubbish. I always told customers there was nothing in these new computer things. The company has gone out of business now.

---

[15] The main premises of Norfolk County Council; the author's employer at time of writing.

[16] A UK high street retail chain that occasionally leases floor space to other companies providing specialist services.

[17] A two year study period at school after the end of compulsory education at age 16. Students work to obtain qualifications that allow entry to University, and often have a part-time job to earn spending money.

While at University I worked for a company called Running Buffet. As the name indicates, they provided catering for events such as birthdays, art openings, and many others in venues around London. These were held in museums, galleries, and the like. I drove the van. It sounds good, doesn't it? But I was also in charge of all the wine. That was like putting Adolf Hitler in charge of a synagogue. It was a total disaster. I lived with three other lads in Richmond at the time. Somehow I always had to pass our home on the way back to base after an event. Our house rapidly became party land. There were masses of free food and wine. It's probably why I've drunk so much wine since. The company has gone out of business now.

After my time at University, I worked for the Royal Bank of Scotland on the overseas trading desk. I am sure that the current world's economic disaster cannot be all down to me. I admit I was more interested in the sexy young secretary who was listening to my Psychology chat up lines than concentrating on my job, but I'm sure Sri Lanka and Sierra Leone are one and the same place, aren't they? Close enough, anyway. The worldwide banking community collapsed, and had to be bailed out. They didn't go out of business. Not quite.

Then I was offered a job as a Corrections Officer at Wandsworth Prison. We should all be grateful I did not take up that position. Fast forward from there to fulltime work and fulltime failure.

In the late 1980's I started working for Tarmac as a Quantity Surveyor[18]. I had left University with a Bsc Hons degree in History and Psychology. This new career was chosen for me by my bank manager. My degree might have been pathetic, but my £10,000 overdraft was something to behold. So Tarmac sent me to Wolverhampton Polytechnic to obtain a qualification in Quantity Surveying. My fellow inmates hated me immediately. I was earning £15,000 per annum while they were all losing a similar amount. My digs were in Wendsfield. I soon learnt that the name 'Wendsfield' is Old Saxon English for "the lowest dung hole in the universe where even the cockroaches apply for housing improvement schemes". As I entered the mud hut that was to be my new home, the first thing I noticed was the other resident - a huge cannabis plant. When I ventured out of the hut, I was a showstopper. The rioting ceased. The locals tried to decide what to do with me, but given that I am white, I was clearly not of their planet or part of the great race war that was going on. So they just let me wander around a bit.

Having survived living and studying in Wolverhampton, I worked as a Quantity Surveyor in various parts of

---

[18] 'A very boring job that has something to do with buildings' - The Author to Editor in conversation.

London. I was also involved in the construction of the Welwyn Garden City shopping centre. Given that I was the new boy, and that God hates me, I always ended up with the scaffolding and steel erecting packages. Now, I will not deny that scaffolding and steel erecting takes great skill and experience, but, along with these talents, there is also another requirement: a history of GBH[19]. Now, the specific duties of a Quantity Surveyor involve robbing subcontractors on a job of their money. I was a 5'7" bespectacled, balding, unfit man, whose most violent action ever has been a rather significant fart. Typically, they would be a gang of 6'3" murdering apes who ate babies for breakfast. And I had to face them and tell them they could not have their rape, pillage and murder tokens. I was always useless as a Quantity Surveyor, but fantastic at dodging fire extinguishers.

In the end, Tarmac realised that my hospital expenses were outstripping the money I was saving them. So they decided to lose me somewhere. In fact, they buried me under the English Channel for two and half years. It might sound great to be involved in such an iconic project as the Channel Tunnel, but a bloody large hole remains a bloody large hole no matter how many times you go down it. There was nothing fantastic about the job. In fact, all I can remember about it now is sleeping in an old army camp and ingesting vast quantities of egg

---

[19] Grievous Bodily Harm - a term used in English criminal law.

and chips. Apart from being stripped naked by a lady darts team and a dubious romantic liaison with a female employee of MacDonalds in Dover. I was made redundant straight after leaving the project.

What was I to do next? Instead of putting my obvious talents at working behind a bar to good use, I decided to teach. Unlike a real educator, I ended up teaching Maths, English and Life Skills at Feltham Young Offenders Institute. To be honest, I did enjoy it, but I was faced every day with a room full of boys whose parents had decided that mature parenting meant giving them everything they asked for to shut them up. Or, if they had nothing to give, then a good kicking was an adequate substitute.

The result was that these kids had no real idea of a strong and fair parent. They had not been brought up to know love or common sense and so they sought that strength from others in similar circumstances. Add a nice dollop of crime to the mix, and the vast availability of money from drugs and surprise, surprise – a whole generation of lost causes. Put them all together in one place so they can learn from each other the one thing they had not learnt yet; how to expand their crime spree.

My job was to stop that. Obviously, none of them had any academic qualifications. I was to provide them with the basics to pass those exams, the genius idea being that they would use them to gain employment. Such employment likely to be a minimum wage of, say £200 a week in a factory or an office. On the other hand, they could go out and earn a minimum of £200 a night selling drugs. And these kids are all under the age of 18. So guess what the success rate was like? I had less chance of success than there was of Margaret Thatcher becoming Arthur Scargill's lover.[20]

But I did learn a few things. When facing a classroom like this, you identify the most vocal guy and completely humiliate him. Unfortunately, he's also likely to be the biggest, and, as our Almighty Creator made me a midget and a weakling, that was a bit of a problem. All I had was my fine ability at bullshit and many changes of underwear. But I never had to call the guards in. I am proud of that. There was only one fight, and thankfully I discovered the value of placing a well-aimed chair into a kid's kneecap. Most of what I taught was not on the curriculum, of course, and God help us all if the lessons had been recorded as they probably are now.

They learnt fractions easily. Well, you have to know how to divide up the drugs, don't you? When it came to ratios, we practised using the gears of cars. Cars and the joyriding of them was a hobby of many of my students so they could see the value of such knowledge. I found

---

[20] Bitterly opposed political figures in the UK in the 1980s. Both thought by some to be mad.

similar examples for other parts of the curriculum. Most of the English course was based around what one says in a courtroom, or how to plough through the bureaucracy of the benefits system. I also had to teach Life Skills. Before you ask, I never really knew what they were either. How to do up your shoelaces I guess. But I took it to mean aggression control, which was always going to be a problem for them when being arrested and then dealing with solicitors. I sincerely hope the legal profession thanks me for this little bit of work I did on their behalf.

Out of this, and all the other work I did in workshops for those at risk in Wandsworth, there is only one success that I know about. I managed to get one guy interested in his future and saving his arse. To begin with, I employed him as my housekeeper. Of course, I was exploiting a source of cheap labour, but during this time I got him an interview for a job in the construction trade. My old work colleagues still thought I was a nice guy even if my personal assessment of my previous career was less than stellar. Well, the young lad got the job and off he went. Some six to nine months later, I was almost assaulted in the local supermarket by his mother. She flung her arms around me thanking me for everything and insisting that my ability to walk on water was really rather good. Nice, but a public embarrassment and untrue. I only did the above. Ok, there was some extra study to help him pass his exams. But he did it himself, and that's the fact. That was what that job taught me. A person has to want to make a change. Otherwise, everything you do for them is a waste of time. The lad's mother had also seen the benefits of good parenting, or possibly the negative effect of her relationship with her partner. Whether she shot the boy's father or not, I have no idea, of course. However, it was one of the few moments in my life that I felt I had done something worthwhile, or assisted in it, at least.

I left Feltham after about two and a half years when I was told by a wife to be that I needed money. Like a moron, I always do what a woman tells me to do. Ok, I agree; mostly it is wise, particularly if you have no real sensible idea of what you want to do in life. But I will always miss that job.

There is one question that arose out of all this prison work that's always left me baffled. Why telling someone that you had sexual intercourse with their mother should cause such an outburst of grief. Especially when it's obviously untrue. Especially amongst those whose mothers who were a waste of space at the very best. I remain stumped. Good luck to anyone who wants to try and insult me that way. My mother is 75 years old and that whole scenario is simply never going to happen. Perhaps my indifference has something to do with my level of self-confidence. Perhaps other people's lack of it is why they have a problem with pointless insults. That, I feel, is the main issue that drives a wide range of people into stupid behaviour. But, as I said earlier, this is not a book about counselling.

So what happened to me next? Obviously, I walked down the street, into an emlpoyment bureau and got a job with the Foreign Office.[21]

All very logical. It was quite literally as simple as that. I went full time with them a year later. To do that, I had to pass the Foreign Office civil service exam. That was very tough. The year I applied there were 2,000 candidates for every available place. So, how was I to manage, I hear those who doubt my intelligence cry out. Well, I knew a number of people who had taken the exams before, so I sat with them and we went through old papers together. When I sat the exam, it turned out to be one that I had already worked on. I passed. Lots of people failed. Those who did not apply tactics, or cheat.

This great epic period of my working life started rather well, albeit a little off the wall as usual. The Foreign Office employed me because I knew about finance. I was given the Conference Department's budget to look after. It was worth £30 million. There was another chap involved. He was not from the Foreign Office but em-

---

[21] The Foreign and Commonwealth Office (FCO), commonly called 'The Foreign Office'; a department of UK Government. Its main responsibility is to protect and promote British interests worldwide.

ployed by another government department. He allegedly had some idea of finance. I never saw that part of his talents. A recently graduated student chef was with us for a while too but left. (Anyone found making jokes about 'cooking the books' will be severely beaten).

So off we went; running the Commonwealth Heads of Summit, Asia, the G8, and the European summit of 1997-1998. Despite the obvious weakness in financial management, we remained within budget for all of the conferences.

Excuse me, but I must digress for a moment. Some lunatic woman has just phoned with the news that my separated wife is marrying someone in Albania in February. Of course, a normal conversation one expects at home on a Wednesday evening. I wonder what the heck is going on with that? There is no rest when you're an 'Unlucky Bastard'. It's a full-time job. I suppose it serves me right for showing off in the paragraph above.

To return to my diplomatic career. All went well at the start. I met lots of famous people. I was never smiled at by Tony Blair, despite his ridiculous smile for everyone else. Maybe that man knew something after all. There are many events I could talk about here, but this is supposed to be a dissertation on the cumulative effects of stupidity more than anything else. So I will restrict the silliness to a minimum. Besides, lots of the happenings are as simple as "I was the man in the lift who pressed the button to the 4th floor for Nelson Mandela". Not exactly exciting, I agree, so let's pick a few with some meat on.

Clinton has a reputation for being a bit smutty. At the G8 Summit, I was looking after the computers. Yes, I have no idea how that potential catastrophe was overlooked either, but there I was. The doors to the office suddenly opened and in walked the most powerful man in the world. Trust me, that description is bullshit. I have been a high-level civil servant and politicians are just annoying flies in the ointment. They are not in charge. Anyway, even though it wasn't part of the inspection route he was supposed to take, there he was: President Clinton.

I was the only member of the Foreign Office in the room and was forced into immediate, diplomatic conversation. Thank God neither of us had any idea about computers so we just bullshitted. I introduced my team as they arrived back from various jobs nearby. Then the nightmare. One girl was doing an errand for me in another part of the building. The computer area was heavily air-conditioned, so we all wore white shirts or blouses. Oh dear. The girl ran back in and gave me the message she'd been sent for. Then she looked into the eyes of the President of United States of America who was standing next to me. Unfortunately, both his eyes and mine were firmly fixed on her very erect nipples, which were caused by the sudden change in temperature. There was a photograph taken of President Clinton and Mr. Griffith together. We are both staring at a young woman's tits. Thank God, it was never printed. Clinton did smile at me and we shook hands afterwards.

Then I went to the toilet. Now this would seem an innocent thing for anyone to do, even at a conference full of various very important people. I was standing there with my rather personal equipment in my hand when BASH WHAM - the door is almost kicked down by three very large blokes. They are followed by a very pissed Famous World Leader[22]. Now, I have been drunk on more than one occasion in my life but this was something else. Famous World Leader was a lost cause; unable to stand; dribbling; a spaced out look on his face. He was trying to speak but he was not using a language indigenous to his native land. Or probably any other.

He was hurled into a cubicle with one of his toilet specialists. One big injection and a few bad noises later and bingo! A minute later he is back in action. Stone cold sober. Then a senior member of the Foreign Office entered the toilet to tell me that I had seen nothing at all. But what a super cure that injection must be if you've had a massive amount too many on a Friday night. I

_____

[22] This name has been omitted on legal advice.

reckon there have been times that many of us could have done with a quick shot of it! What remains a mystery to me is how did the man manage to get so drunk, and just how did his team explain it to the other world leaders around the table? Talk about an inappropriate time to get plastered. This incident is one of the few examples I can give you where there was someone worse off than me.

I had another opportunity to showcase my natural diplomatic abilities at a major conference. I was surrounded by Presidents and Prime Ministers. Security was everywhere. Jesus, it looked like a bloody Blues Brothers reunion. I was in charge of one little area. And lo, suddenly in front of me, in my corridor there appeared four scruffy tarts. Where the hell had they come from? It was my duty to send them back to the filth where they belonged. So I told them to f**k off out of it. Then I noticed that there were TV cameras and photographers all around these little street urchins. I'd never heard of the female band All Saints.[23] Fortunately, the camera crew also thought they were tossers, and I was saved from any public humiliation. I believe that the group has died a death now anyway.

There were a few other odd jobs I did before the Foreign Office sent me overseas. Guess what they left me in

---

[23] An all girl English-Canadian pop group who sold approximately 11 million records worldwide including 5 number one singles in the UK.

control of? Nuclear weapons. Now you feel really safe, do you not? In reality, it meant keeping an eye on where the little Greenpeace idiots were in the world in relation to our rather large 'piss off' nuclear submarines. And making sure they did not meet. I also got to write questions and answers for the Foreign Secretary. As I am sure you may have guessed, none of the stuff you see on TV is unrehearsed in the House of Commons[24]. All the Members know what is coming to them as a question, and the answer that they will give. They also know the next question after that, and the appropriate response. And so on. So this is democracy. A whole load of civil servants writing it all out for the elected representatives of the people to recite parrot fashion for the populace to listen to. I trust everyone is happy with this!!

There are an endless multitude of jobs in the civil service as I have indicated. That helps to explain why every letter you get back from them is basically the same. Just full of bullshit words created for a bit of a laugh to send out to the poor population of the country that pay for civil servants to sit there and make up bloody stupid long sentences that mean nothing and result in nothing ever happening.

However, in the Foreign Office, there is the chance to be a total lunatic overseas. Oh, joy! You do not have to

---

[24] The elected lower house of parliament of the United Kingdom.

have any specific talent, but you are told that you are representing our fine and honourable Queen and country. In my case, mostly from the other end of a bottle of dubious-tasting wine.

In the year 2000, I arrived at a shack that was allegedly the international airport at Sofia in Bulgaria. I drove through the streets from the terminal. They were lined with the many shacks where the people lived. I arrived at the office at the Embassy. It was a shack. The whole Embassy was a shack.

My job was dealing with emmigration and consular work. Big surprise; in 2000, all the Bulgarians wanted to leave Bulgaria. I dealt with thousands upon thousands of these idiots. Hundreds said they were plumbers and builders, but their only working experience was behind various bars. Mostly located in shacks with no toilets. One applicant even changed his name to Manchester United and told the UK press about it. Why do that? So I would believe that he was going to return to his shack after attending a football game in the UK. Never mind that the match ticket would cost him 15 years of his regular income. As you will appreciate, the refusal rate for application was very, very high. You had more chance of surviving the first wave of the July 1st, 1916 assault at the Somme than getting a visa in those circumstances. All this resulted in my being on the wrong end of many gipsy curses, which, it turns out, may have had something to them after all!

Work as Vice-Consul in Bulgaria was not particularly onerous, most of it was actually rather straightforward. It was 2004 and the miserable folk we call holidaymakers had not discovered the country yet. There was no tide of Brits, eager to obtain an STD as a memento of their visit. But there were a few of my fellow countrymen there at the time. Most of them wanted to buy property. Here's what usually happened. Mr. & Mrs. Brit would arrive at a bar in deepest Bulgaria with 20,000 Euros in a little bag. That kind of behaviour is the equivalent of turning up in a backstreet pub in the UK with £250,000 in used bank notes. The conversation would go something like this:

Mr. & Mrs. Mad Brit: "We like that little place on the hill. Does anyone know who owns it?"
Little Bulgarian Man: "Well, it is mine."
Mr. & Mrs. Mad Brit: "That's lucky. We wish to buy it with this bag of money."
Little Bulgarian Man: "Ok. I will sign this piece of paper so you can have the house."
Mr. & Mrs. Mad Brit: "Brilliant. Here is the bag of money. We will go home now to collect our things."

On their return a couple of weeks later, the bar is all closed up. Everyone has gone. Oh, well, not to worry.

They go to the house. And find a family sat down to dinner in their own home. What a shock! That was when they would come running to me, screaming because they had lost all their money. Of course, no solicitor had been involved at any stage. How can you really sympathise with people as stupid as that?

There were a few brave tourists who ventured that far into Europe back then and one of my responsibilities was to provide them with helpful literature and information. More often, I did the same for the many British ministers and trade delegations who visited on official and political business. One of these pieces of literature was a street map of Sofia, produced annually by the Office of the City Mayor. I had been handing out these maps for quite a while before someone noticed that there were little love hearts all over them. "Oh, how romantic of the Mayor!" I thought. For about a second. Until the cold, horrifying realisation dawned on me. For the previous six months, I had been supplying all the visiting British dignitaries with specific directions to every illegal brothel in the city. Including the one that was next door to the Ambassador's residence. How did I know? Trust me, we all knew.

I actually fell off the back of a lorry when I was there. A British Army friend and I were with a party skiing in the mountains. When we went to return, his car had broken down. Being the gentlemen we were, we insisted that everyone else go back in the other vehicles. We would remain and wait for help. True, there was a rather nice pub nearby with some rather nice waitresses, but it's the thought that counts. The breakdown truck arrived and the car was pushed up onto the back of it. Suddenly, I realised that I'd left my coat on the passenger seat. I climbed up the side of the lorry and opened the car door. It is a little-known fact that car doors open outwards. I stepped back into thin air and fell seven feet onto solid ice. I hurt my back and bruised my ribs. However, Bulgarian wine served by rather nice waitresses is a good form of pain relief. They did laugh at me for several hours, though.

Another British Army friend was a chap called Karl. He was a delightful bloke; very polite, handsome, and dedicated to his job. He was also quite a hit with the ladies. I have no idea why he wanted to hang out with me. He met my sister once. She squirted the contents of a coffee percolator into his crotch. I don't remember if he had much interest in women after that. But he was still athletic and purchased a self-assembly indoor gym kit. He was living in the shack above mine at the time so he gave me a call and asked me to help him set it up. Yes, you read that correctly. A member of the British Army asked me to help him put together some gym equipment. Now, I have never been inside a gym in my life, and never will, let alone actually interact with the instruments of torture within.

Worse was to come. His diplomatic bag was filled with his monthly supply of port and cheese. These were items of great value in Bulgaria, where the only really edible thing was the caviar. And, believe me, after four years of caviar, you hate it in any form. Good quality port and a fairly wide variety of cheese were like nectar in those circumstances. The idea was to savour them for a month or so until another order made it out to us. I arrived at his flat at about 9 pm. At 10 am the following morning, the gym kit remained in pieces. Only I was draped over it like a soldier in no man's land; caught on the barbed wire and dying slowly. Karl was crashed out on the sofa. A month's golden supply of port and cheese was lying discarded all around us. I was never invited back.

One evening I was just finishing work when the phone rang. I had been heading home, or to another bar, but the call was from a woman in the UK trying to trace the whereabouts of her brother. Normally, this would just have involved taking down all the details, which I did, of course. The thing was that I knew who she was talking about. He was a drunk who had died bankrupt at the beach on the other side of the country some years before. We had sent details to the UK police at the time, of course, but they had been unable to trace any family. As a result, he had been buried in an unmarked, pauper's grave.

Now, as it had taken four years to look him up, it was obvious they were not a close family. So, you would have thought that confirmation of his passing would have been enough. Oh, no. The whole family decided to come over for a holiday and visit the grave to pay their respects.

So I head over to the other side of the country in advance of their arrival. I get to the cemetery. There are bloody thousands of dead people there, and hundreds of unmarked graves. My feeble enquiries fail to find one dead English drunk buried four years earlier. Hardly surprising. But his sister, an aunt, an uncle, and a couple of other relatives are already en route. The British Consul, the Embassy Vicar, and an English/Bulgarian translator are all on their way as well. I was only missing one thing: the corpse. There was only one solution. I randomly picked one of the unmarked graves and had it cleaned up. So, everyone arrived and paid their final respects. Probably to Boris the Bulgarian, or someone's pet cat.

Bulgaria is known for its mafia connections. But, they weren't a great problem for us. They mostly kept to themselves. They were just large stupid gorillas with guns who wanted money and women. So long as you didn't run into a Russian member, you were fine. However, we still had to keep an ear out for possible trouble. Part of my duties meant looking after the emergency phone 24/7 for three weeks at a time. The very first evening I was doing this, I happened to be in a bar. All my mates kept on ringing me up with ridiculous questions. A lot of these involved one of my ex-wives. They knew I had to answer the phone, of course. I had no choice.

After a while, I started to get pretty annoyed. One call even claimed to be from the Canadian Embassy in Bucharest of all places! Someone asking if any foreign nationals had been killed in the bomb explosion in the centre of Sofia. I think my response of "Look, just f**k off, will you?" was perfectly rational in the circumstances. Almost at once, a hush fell over the bar. I looked around, desperately trying to locate the potential joker. It was me. I had just told the Canadian Consul to f**k off. There had been a bomb explosion in the city, and there were unknown numbers of casualties. The good news was that the dead and maimed were all members of the Bulgarian mafia. The bad news was the little chat that I had to have with the Ambassador the next day. So much for Bulgaria.

My next posting was to Eketeringberg in Siberia. The Foreign Office hated me. The place is famous for the assassination of the Tsar and his family. That is it. Well, that and being minus 40 degrees centigrade in the winter. But I was all set with my long johns and polar expedition gear. Almost at once, I was posted to Sudan, where it's plus 40 degrees centigrade. All the bloody time. I was left standing in the desert in my winter thermals.

There are only two words to sum up my tour in Sudan — hot and violent. In the mid-2000s, the South and North regions were one country, although there was fighting all the time. Weekend entertainment was watching university students being hit with tear-gas, and army trucks shooting at people as they passed by. In Egypt, you saw a dead horse in a ditch and thought nothing of it. In Sudan, you saw a dead student in a ditch and thought nothing of it.

Khartoum is the capital of Sudan. It was extremely Muslim. All women were covered from head to toe, with only their eyes visible, and were not allowed to talk to any man. Alcohol was not permitted. All this on pain of death from the authorities. Obviously, I ended up with a nymphomaniac for a maid and in charge of the only bar in the entire country.

The nymphomaniac maid was an easy mistake to make. Anyone could have done it. The fine Welsh Baptist Security Officer at the Embassy introduced me to her. He told me that she was a good, young Christian girl who could do all my cleaning and cooking for me. He knew her family well. She turned up at my house and said very little. She had a slight build and dark eyes, but I could tell little else. Christian or not, we were in the North of the country so she was fully clothed, albeit not as covered up as the Muslim women. Day two, and the first thing she did when she arrived was stick her tongue down my throat. I don't pretend to be familiar with all the forms of greeting in the world, but this was a little more informal than I expected.

Naturally, I had to terminate her employment, although it did take three months for me to make certain that this greeting, and everything that followed, was just a mistake. It took time to confirm all the facts, you understand. The final straw was not the obvious risk of disease or fear of discovery and subsequent death from the authorities. In fact, it involved the Embassy Maintenance Officer. While we were talking, he got a call on his mobile. He refused the request the caller was making. Two seconds later, my phone rang. It was the maid, asking for more money and an advance on her salary. I refused. The Maintenance Officer and I never discussed what happened. You can be friends with someone, share a meal, and share an office. But there are some things that you just can't share. Good Christian maids being one of them. After that two male security guards cooked and cleaned for me. I have never lived in such a clean place, or (God Bless, Mum) had such well-ironed shirts. I taught them English, and we had some very nice meals together.

The bar was a situation sent straight from my best mate God. I do not know why the British Embassy was the only place allowed to serve alcohol in Sudan, but we were. Perhaps it was something to do with them taking General Gordon's head? I have no idea. My job was Senior Management Officer. I was in complete charge. Similar unlikely events include Stalin and Hitler making a pact of non-aggression over Poland in 1939. The world was stunned. Better still, there was a beautiful pool right next to it. One walked out of the bar with one's cocktail, sat down, and dangled one's feet in the pool. Delightful. There are only two types of weather in Sudan; bloody hot and pink sandstorm. Bloody hot equalled sitting by the pool and pink sandstorm equalled sitting in the cool, air-conditioned bar.

The place was only open to the public on a Thursday. This was 'guest night' and when the weekend really started. I was allowed half a dozen guests in my own right, as were all the other Embassy staff. However, I had the final approval on those as well. I could also use the invites allocated to any member of staff who had not invited someone. They might be away, or they did not go to the bar, or they had no friends. Perhaps they were so boring that they could not even purchase friends by way of those invites. It was a very democratic system (for me, anyway). As a result, the bar would be swarming every Thursday with horny little Scandinavians, Irish, Italians, Dutch, and so on. These were all lovely little people who were making their contribution to the world by working for the United Nations and various international voluntary groups. Of course, there were far more Americans than any other nationality in the country at that time. But, as far as I know, they were all tee-total, because none of them ever made it into the bar. How odd is that? Perhaps, God is actually an American, and the situation that I find myself in now is his revenge upon me!

I never had so many friends in my life as when I ran that bar, especially when each week crawled toward a Thursday night. I was a very popular young chap. Unless you happened to be an American, I suppose. The only time we had a problem was the evening of my leaving party. I opened the bar up to everyone on that occasion, including the locals. Now, we were paid more than enough on those 'hardship postings', particularly as spouses were not allowed to come along. So, I was not as generous as you might think when I put a load of money behind the bar. It's what I did at main events, anyway. In all the different embassies I worked at, it was always the locals who ran the ship. And they deserved to be rewarded for all their hard work.

However, as you will remember, Sudan was a place where no alcohol was allowed. So, it was obvious what happened. Did everyone remain sane and sensible, and spend all night drinking fruit juice, or whatever their various religious laws dictated? Or did they all get totally and utterly pissed and start tribal fighting that security had to sort out? Did we then have to run a gauntlet of local police to get them all home safe before anyone smelt alcohol on their breath? Please guess. My conversation with the Ambassador the following morning was not pleasant.

I shall return to the bar in a little while, as I always do, although the circumstances will be somewhat different. This posting did give me the opportunity to meet some very famous people. When I first arrived, I was quartered at the best hotel in Khartoum, while my residential accommodation was being sorted out. The management gave me a suite by the pool, either because I was a very important guest, or because I was the only nutter who would drink the vile Sudanese coffee without sugar.

One morning I was sitting on my veranda, wondering if what the street cat had managed to catch was more edible than my breakfast. The only way to eat the shit food was to deaden the taste buds with the unsweetened coffee. A few feet away from me on the neighbouring veranda was a black guy. I had no idea who he was so I just struck up a conversation, warning him to be careful with the coffee. It could probably kill, after all. Inevitably, we got around to why he was in Sudan. As I've said, the country was in turmoil at the time and there were lots of diplomats trying to place band aids over the whole sorry mess. As we were talking, all the briefings we'd been having over the previous month came to mind and the truth suddenly dawned on me. I was talking to United Nations General Secretary, Kofi Annan.

It was too late by then, but we just carried on. Two blokes having a chat over the shared nightmare of an inedible breakfast in a dung hole of a country. By then I'd noticed the massive entourage of people hanging around in the background, and some seriously well-armed guards. I couldn't help but mention how the cost-cutting Foreign Office had assigned me two little lads with twigs to do the same job that half a dozen fully armed combat troops were doing for him. Those were the same two lads who went on to clean and cook for me later on. The ones that I taught English. Kofi's armed guards were Americans. They are still illiterate.

Despite Kofi being a nice chap, it all went wrong in Sudan and the country eventually ended up splitting in two. But many things went on during those times that were barely reported in the Western media. The President of South Sudan was supposed to be sharing power with his Northern counterpart in the role of his deputy. This arrangement was intended to give the southern region greater autonomy. A few weeks after this arrangement was made, he set out for Khartoum to take up his appointment. He disappeared on the way. The news broke that he had been killed in a helicopter crash. Now, as you may recall, I mentioned that weekends in the capital were spent watching riots. Well, this was a whole new ball game. We went straight from the Conference League to the Premier.[25] This was civil war. And God loved me so much, he decided that it was all going to kick off on the day that I was supposed to be flying home. Of course. What else could happen to me?

Unless you are a dedicated historian, you probably don't realise that civil wars are not fought by two sides alone. The English Civil War, for example, was not just contested by Cavaliers and Roundheads. There were many other groups right across the political spectrum that were involved. The American Civil War is another case in point. The Sudanese uprising of 2005 was no different. There are a multitude of religious groups in the country, not just Christian and Muslim, and also countless tribes with their own affiliations. All were represented in the rank and file of the National Army and the Police Force, both groups being gathered in Khartoum at the time, awaiting the arrival of the new Vice-President.

Then the news came through that he was dead. Everyone suspected it was no accident. The students went out on 'strike' and onto the streets. Mainly to fight. As they always did. The really bad news was that the army split

---

[25] The English Football League. The Premier League features such teams as Chelsea and Manchester United, the National Conference teams such as Torquay United and Solihull Moors.

into two factions and started shooting at each other. The police joined in, followed by any civilian who fancied it. So, there I was, sitting in my office when it all kicked off, wondering if I had a spare pair of underpants.

You can't just abandon an embassy. A fleet of helicopters doesn't just drop you at the airport and it's back to Blighty for tea and crumpets. That only happens in American movies. Evacuation in such extreme circumstances is a serious business. The only saving grace was that neither side had declared war on Britain. But some of the factions certainly weren't going to be in love with us, so the Embassy was a potential target. And the trouble would be coming our way eventually.

As you may remember, I mentioned before that it's the local staff that run the Embassy. There were about 200 of them. They all lived outside the centre of the city, in homes that had armed guards and wouldn't be known to the mob anyway. So, getting most of them evacuated out of the firing line wasn't difficult. However, some were working away from the Embassy that day, and others had children attending local schools. So I sent out all the vehicles we had to try and bring them back.

They returned in dribs and drabs. I handed out paper and pencils and did my best to play the father figure to the kids. Our drivers were amazing. They avoided all the grief that was quickly spreading through the city and got everyone back to the Embassy. I arranged minibuses out of the city to get them all back to their homes. It's probably the only thing I can be proud of in my pathetic little life.

During all this, I was helped by a young English lad, who rode a motorbike. I don't remember his name, but his cool head was very handy to have in a crisis. Just as the last of the staff were leaving, my phone rang. It was the British Council, who had offices almost next door.: "Mark, what do we do? The rioters are burning our cars outside the building, and we are stuck on the roof. Help us!" To be honest, they always were a bunch of wankers. Obviously, all I had to do was go to the front gate and ask everyone politely to stop. They were only civilians with weapons. And members of the police and armed forces. Well, I told them to leave it me, and somehow we got through it. No one was hurt, and there was no real damage inflicted on the building or the people, just a couple of torched cars.

There are certain protocols and procedures to follow in such a situation. The Embassy must be 'locked down'. So I abandoned my office and set up temporary headquarters elsewhere. In the bar. The sole representative of the British Embassy in Khartoum and not feeling very Victorian about it all. And then I realised something. Undoubtedly, my organisation of the evacuation had been a work of genius. But I had forgotten one thing: me. My own arse was now seriously hanging out.

So, dear reader, please picture this real life scene. A balding man in a suit sat by a pool with a glass of wine in one hand, and a cigarette in the other. Rifle fire moving steadily closer, and the screams and yelling of the mob getting louder. The noise of tank fire and machine guns in the distance. My phone rings. I am saved! No, it's my wife. She's demanding that I pick up as many large-size tampons as possible when I'm in London before I fly out to my next posting. I try to explain that I'm in the middle of a civil war and likely to die. I apologise in advance in case the tampons did not arrive. But she just goes on and on and on. I've not had the best of luck with wives, but this really was the pits. It was impossible for her not to hear the gunfire, especially as I took the phone outside to emphasise the point that our conversation might have to wait until a more convenient time. She just hung up.

While I stood there considering tampons and the fact that my life was about to end, a van pulled up. It was the Ambassador's driver. There are few times in my life when I have achieved absolute joy. That was one of them. He told me that we had a mission. Go back to my own residence, pick up my stuff, and go to the airport so I can catch a plane and leave. It was a mission I chose to accept.

It was the first time, and I hope the last, that I have travelled through a war zone. To some extent, it looked like it does in the movies. There were burnt-out cars, buildings in flames, and dead bodies. But people don't get shot or burnt to death in a nice way, so I'll spare you the gruesome details. Apart from to note that it doesn't matter what colour you may be before you burn, everyone is the same colour afterwards.

As we headed through the streets, I learnt something else; my stupid British Diplomatic Passport did not stop bullets. There was a sudden clatter of shots. One of then hit the van with an awfully solid clunk. The driver looked at me. 'What now, Mr. Mark?' 'Just fuck off quick,' I replied. He understood. I think they were just warning shots that went wrong, but, when I looked back down the road, I saw a tank.

Eventually, we made it to my house. The protection detail was still in place. Yes, the two guys with twigs had not abandoned their post. Very good of them, but also very stupid. Or was it? I gave them half of all the money that I had left on me. The driver already had the other half, along with my promise to marry his sister, I think. We made it to the airport. Unbelievably, there was a plane due in shortly that would take me away. I made my farewells to what remained of my staff and handed over my phone.

There was an American in the waiting room, and another guy from somewhere in Europe. There was a big sign that said 'Do Not Smoke.' We all lit up and stood together under it. There is a tank at the end of the runway. The European wasn't taking it so hard. He knew that the American would be shot first if it came to that. The American smelled of fouled underpants. After a couple of hundred years, the plane arrived. It's wasn't much of an aircraft, but it had wings and it moved. No one shot at us as we took off.

By now, I have missed all my original flight connections, of course, and the plane landed somewhere else in Africa anyway. But at least, it was a place where everyone wasn't trying to kill each other. Or me. Eventually, I made it back to London. My family were expecting me three days earlier. Remember, I had no phone. Sensibly, they'd contacted the Foreign Office to ask what had happened to me. Their response? That I had left on time and they had no idea. Bloody useless!

As a postscript to these events, you'll be pleased to learn that I did pick up a load of extra-large absorbent tampons in London. A few days later, I filled up my hand luggage with them and headed off to my next posting in Albania. I was stopped at Gatwick and had to open the case in front of everyone.

My next assignment, then: Albania. Another Muslim state. Except, in practice, it isn't. In fact, the religious mix of the country is mostly Christian Orthodox, Muslim and Coffee Cup Reading. The 'Muslim' designation is down to the Turks, who ran the country for 500 years. It was a deal they offered the population; change your name, be a Muslim, and we'll cut your taxes. So everyone did. A no-brainer. The good news for yours truly, of course, was that most everyone smoked and drank. What the Albanians do believe in I don't know, unless it's attempting to make money quickly without working, and talking a lot about it afterwards. That's not everyone in the country, of course. I excuse my father-in-law and one friend of mine. But that's it. No matter how nice they may seem, the rest of them have brains from another planet.

I doubt that you've ever been to Albania so I am sure you all want to know what the country is like. Well, allow me to be explicit. It's a SHITHOLE. Hardly surprising that everyone wants to leave. Remember what I said about Bulgaria when I was there in 2000? That was a paradise, compared to Albania. My job when I was there? Visa officer. It was simple really: "No, your visa is refused."

To give you an idea, I'm going to quote you some figures from my famous court case (more of which in a later chapter). In 2007, the average percentage of UK Visa applications that were refused from across the world was 6%. This statistic includes Western Europe, the USA, Canada, Australia and New Zealand. The average refusal rate for Eastern Europe was 26%. But the refusal rate posted by Mr. Bastard Griffith in Albania was 84%. I was the biggest refusal merchant in the entire world. And some of the 16% that did get past me were those on ministerial visits on behalf of the Albanian government and professionals such as airline pilots (and they only got a work permit!)

The Albanian politicians were like something from a children's TV programme. They shouted for joy, they cried, they had no idea. Tirana is the capital city. It needed rebuilding. The people were living in concrete blocks. The Mayor's solution? Paint all the concrete blocks.

Actually, I liked the rough and ready attitude of some of their elected officials, but the vast majority of them were so full of bull, it was almost unbelievable. The country will never change until the next generation takes over. My Albanian sister-in-law is an architect, but it will take many more like her before anything gets done. At the moment, the general population mostly live in villages. They are very proud of their villages. Some are proud that their village has the best potatoes. This is serious.

But there is more to see in Tirana than in Khartoum. Khartoum has a couple of blokes spinning around like my 2-year old son. They are called the dervishes. It has some mini black pyramids in the middle of the desert. It has a line in two rivers which indicates where the White and the Blue Nile meet.

Tirana also has a river. It flows through the middle of the city like an open sewer. Tirana has a small restaurant on a tower that turns around so you can be continually depressed with a 360-degree view of the place where the Foreign Office has sent you. There are a few museums, but an afternoon is sufficient to complete your sightseeing tour. It's also where I met the wife I am currently divorcing.

The countryside is full of some 500,000 bunkers designed to prevent invasion. These were built during the time of the dictator Hoxha. I would have suggested an advertising campaign promoting Albania as a holiday destination instead. It would have cost a fraction of the amount and have been a far greater deterrent to the march of Imperialism. The roads are what we would call potholes. Many of the population have BMWs stolen from overseas but don't know how to drive them. I read somewhere that they'd only be allowed private motor cars for about 15 years before my arrival, and that they'd been taught to drive by the Greeks and the Italians. The result was total chaos, although their terrible driving did provide an effective birth-control system. I knew three people who died on their roads.

There are 8 million Albanians but when I was there, about half of them were in Greece and Italy. Now that many are being sent home, so I can only imagine what it's like. It's a third world state located in Europe. Yes, I feel sorry for individuals who live there, but not for the population as a whole. They need to learn how to run their country properly or remain the piss-hole of Europe. And I doubt they ever will.

To clarify. Even in the capital, the electricity is only on for part of the time. Whole cities do not pay service bills because they don't have any money. Or because they don't want to. If you stand on a side street in Tirana and look up, you see a mass of wires connected to the electricity and telephone poles. All for the purpose of stealing power from each other. Presumably, all this grand theft ends somewhere with one poor sod paying for it all. Also, the water is undrinkable. I felt somewhat dubious about even washing in it.

I mentioned the roads earlier. Holes and ditches just appeared in them. Repair work was limited. No-one put out cones or tape or barriers. Well, I'm sure you can see where this is going. I was walking back from work one day, talking to my parents on my mobile. They hear a scream, and then silence. At my end, there are a lot of swear words. Suddenly, the ground had disappeared from under my feet and I had dropped six-feet into a drainage ditch. There was only one little lad who was willing to help me. The tip he got was probably the equivalent of a month's pension for his grandfather. Of course, the more cynical amongst you could interpret the situation in a different way. This gipsy kid removed all the warning signs and waited until a victim fell into the hole. Then he helps them out, getting a fat reward in the process. A reward that amounts to a hell of a lot more than he could get from the usual begging.

I am trying to think if anything else remarkable happened to me in Albania, apart from a change of wives. There were nights out and laughs with the friends that I made, of course. There were some good experiences. I have damned the place because that is what should happen to it. But not all of the people should be damned, just 99% of them. Enough of Albania for now. Later on, I will show you its more jovial side.

Finally, we bring my working life right up to date with my current situation. Back in the UK with Norfolk County Council. I started in their Children's Services Department, then moved to Emergency Planning and then Business Support. Let's take a look at my career path there, and the way the All-Powerful One ensured that it got mucked up. It started well. When I was promoted into Emergency Planning, there were strong possibilities of moving up the ladder there. But then another reorganisation was ordered. In one day, I got a pay rise, a pay deduction, was almost made redundant and eventually demoted two grades into the Business Support team.

Well, perhaps I was not so unlucky, after all. I still have a job. My salary will drop, but at least, I held onto the higher rate of pay long enough to secure my home. I can work on the other issues later. Plus if I had gone elsewhere, perhaps another employer would not have been so sympathetic about my current situation. Perhaps they would have just told me to bugger off. And they are not such a bad bunch of eggs to work with. I could be brutally honest about some of them, but I will leave taking the Mickey out of individuals until such time as they have the direct chance of doing the same to me. Otherwise, it just isn't fun. And I must never forget that the good Lord, who has heaped so much misfortune upon me, did throw in a new local pub with this job. And I got to work in it as well.[26]

The only thing that worries me a little about my current job situation are the options to leave on health grounds. There's cancer, stroke, and other serious ailments. Then

---

[26] The Norfolk County Council Staff Sports and Social Club. A membership club that is run and funded entirely by the staff of the County Council. Such socal clubs were often attached to big employers at one time, but this is the sole example remaining in the city of Norwich.

there's pregnancy. Thank you, Lord, for my little piece of manhood. That's one thing I can't get. Adding child-birth to the first option would have been a real drag.

However, before you think that I am going soft and as-suming that my miserable, disgusting life is any more than a long list of unfortunate failures that I am present-ing here to improve your personal sense of well-being, then allow me to detail my wage levels over my work-ing life.

When I was 26 years old in 1992, I was earning a £26,000 basic salary per annum. By the age of around 33 in 1999, this had progressed to £24,000. (I acknowl-edge that various packages like a house, travel, and ex-tras for bad living conditions meant that the money in my pocket was £50,000+ but the basic was 24K). At the age of 45, I was taking home just a basic wage of £24,000 with no extras. Given recent developments and, according to my calculations, at the age 48, I believe my basic salary will be about £18,500. Can anyone spot the obvious problem with my career? Just as well I was never interested in money.

Well, that is the end of my career history. Although, if it's all right with you guys, I would like the chance to bugger up a bit more. A massive cock up that is worthy of note. Trust me, a disaster is pending. I just need the chance!

So what do you guys want next?

Chapter Five: Sex and Marriages

Must be time for the smut by now, eh? You want the full low down on the girls, the sex and marriages? Well, guess what? As the sad man that I am, we can easily sum it all up as follows: it always ended in disaster.

Apart from the specific details of these catastrophes, the only revelation is the actual numbers of women involved. Obviously, three marriages are sufficient to highlight my role as God's Ambassador of Failure. In their own sweet way, all of them are worthy of your attention as a source of humour. But I have had other relationships, and here is my dark secret. I have slept with many women. To be completely honest with you, it cost me a bloody fortune!! No, they weren't all ladies of the night. Not quite, anyway.

So now you have the truth about your little smiley Mark. Perhaps you are revising your opinion of me. If you want me to try to justify it, then please start up a discussion with me some time. You may be interested to know that I stopped all the whorehouses in Sofia from working for three months so drug checks could be carried out. I received a personal commendation from the Chief of Police for that effort. There are many other things of a political and social nature that happened in Bulgaria back then that I could mention. However, they are not part of the history of 'Uber Disaster Man'. In fact, that whole story is a very long and emotional one, and most definitely not for this piece of work.

I have been brutally honest with you in setting the scene, so all that follows may make a little more sense.

One always remembers the first moment of true love. Or, in the case of a 13-year-old boy, the first chance to have sex. We all know from our own bitter experience that it is going to be a disaster. I was with some lass in a village cemetery. To be honest, I'm not sure that either of us received any great revelations from that first sexual experience. What we did receive was gnat bites all over our feet that travelled rapidly upward toward the inevitable areas. The extreme itching and inability to explain it was almost like getting an STD. She, of course, decided that this was God's way of telling us that what we had done was wrong. My personal opinion was that some great gnat festival had been created in the village, and this feasting of many buttocks would never be beheld again. Unfortunately, the buttocks certainly weren't. It took me nine months to recover my position with her after the gnat attack. Trust me, this is a long time when you are 13 or 14-year-old boy. After a short while, she decided that older boys were better anyway. I remember being heart broken and then working out how to get into a similar position again with another young lady. But not, perhaps, in a graveyard.

Like most gentlemen, I made an absolute arse of myself with many delightful young girls. I even followed a Scandanavian girl from Spain to Norway just to be with her. On the way, I met two Danish girls on a train and scored. They decided to turn up in Norwich to spend a week with me. Unfortunately, I was in Norway. Thank god my parents were away at the time. My sister had to look after them. I am told they were very nice. You do the maths, and I think you can work out my big error. I am still paying my sister back for that disaster.

I think overall that my embarrassment at some very, very stupid comments that I have made to women in the past are at least balanced by the fun that I've had. There was one party with eight women and me alone, which will be my final accolade of sexual achievement. It certainly beat blowing the candles out on some lousy cake in front of a load of people who really don't care. It was a rather dramatic change for the usual birthday feast, but I promise you it will never happen again. Honest!

There are a multitude of failed sexual encounters and a long trail of women around this world who are still left wondering what on earth that pathetic little date with the rotund, balding Englishman was all about. However, I think we can leave all of those to your imagination, or perhaps another chapter if requested, and permitted by colleagues in the legal department.

So how about my marriages? I am going to include a warm up relationship before my first marriage. It lasted three years, so I think it qualifies. The easiest way to keep tabs on these relationships is by their religion. They came - and went - in the following order: Catholic, Protestant, Jewish and Muslim.

Catholic: An Irish redhead that I met at University. She was in her last year, and I was in my first. Now, remember, this went on for three years. Never in that entire time did I manage to sleep with this woman. Plenty of others during that period, but never her. I even arranged a holiday on some Greek island for the express purpose. What happened? Her sister came with us. Her sister was not a good-looking redhead. Her sister was a whale. She made ugly a whole new art form and made things even better by being a complete arsehole. Not to be outdone, I invited my sister along. She is good looking, and six foot two inches tall. The holiday went extremely well. For about three minutes. My sister got annoyed with the Whale and decked her with a superb uppercut. My sister and I didn't spend a lot of time with the Redhead and the Whale after that. We had some strange guests over instead. I believe the mess that some of them left behind probably annoyed the Redhead and the Whale. However, they were too polite to say anything. Or perhaps it was the "who gives a fuck" and "by the way my sister is twice your size and will only smack the shit out of you again" attitude that won them over. All in all, it was a rather jolly holiday. I found someone else after that. Albeit eventually.

Protestant: A lovely Welsh girl. I was drunk, and she was available seems to have been the basis for this romance. After a short time the words "marry me" fell out of my mouth. Unfortunately, she heard me, and that was that. Her mother took over all the planning, and despite her small cock up of arranging for my best man, his wife and my family and I to stay in the only brothel in town, I ended up married. We had a lovely roof garden flat in Clapham, which as you can imagine, cost a lot of money. She was a nanny. That did not help our financial circumstances too much. So muggins[27] spent a lot of time working. After a couple of years, I went off to work on the Channel Tunnel project. The money was better, but it meant staying away from home. All was fine. Then I returned home one day to find my wife in bed with another woman. She wasn't even good looking. All was not fine. I went for a quick resolution with my first divorce. This involved handing over a wedge of cash, and wishing them all the best. I was left without a home, furniture and basic essentials. I was soon to learn that this was a way of life.

Jewish: I hadn't had sex for a year, so I married again. God, she was ugly. But I got confused and assumed that

---

[27] Derogatory British term for an idiot, almost always used as a reference to yourself. Origin disputed.

sex meant marriage. She was very organised in many ways, apart from being on time for transport of any kind. That always killed me. She was very keen on my joining the Foreign Office. However, there was a serious problem when we got overseas. Everyone hated her. You have to mix with all sorts of people in the job, and she could mix with none. I was actually offered $10,000 to agree to have her killed in Bulgaria. The offer was 10,000 Euros in Albania. She became a terrible weight around my neck, but relief was at hand. She buggered off with £120,000 of my money.

Muslim: Surely a Muslim would be a good idea? I was led to believe from everyone I knew in Albania, and from my previous posting in Sudan, that Muslim women are subservient to men, and always put their interests first. So I marry one and bang: she turns out to be some kind of revolutionary on her own sweet path of world destruction. All forms of communication are based on levels of screaming. It becomes impossible to plan for the future. Mother-in-law moves in for good, even though we are living in a one bedroom flat with a baby. My life is taken from me. Telephone bills appear that would have beggared belief if they'd emerged from Bletchley Park in the years 1940-1945. Service companies decide they can afford to re-invest in the future of the UK based solely on my quarterly bills. I purchase a larger house on the basis that at least I won't have to sleep with my mother-in-law anymore. My wife loses it by adding physical abuse to the constant screaming. I'd had enough The police were not amused. She lives in a very small flat in London now with her mother and my son.

I have no current plans to marry again.

Chapter Six: Acting

One thing I always loved doing is acting. Thanks to my Mum I had that opportunity from an early age. I have been Pinocchio, a Munchkin and other demanding roles. But from this promising beginning, things took a dark turn, of course. It had to come out in an uber cretin like me.

My next performance of note was on the night I celebrated my 30th year. I stripped completely naked, apart from my socks, while daring a mate with the same date of birth to do the same. He retained his honour, and girlfriend, and keeping his trousers on.

On my 40th birthday, I was in Tirana. I invited numerous Embassy staff and locals to my local restaurant/bar, where I appeared with a real belly dancer. I was all dressed up as well and made a complete arse out of myself and out of our country. I feel that the Ambassador did not take it well. Even if everyone else did.

It was a great hobby but, given current circumstances, it's just as well I did not decide to take it up as a career!! An actor with no voice is a bloody mime artist stuck in a London tube station.

Chapter Seven: Food and Drink

I may not have sampled the available cuisine in every country on the planet, but I have eaten insects in Indochina. Most of the far-flung places I visited were fine; New Zealand, Japan, America, and so on. Europe was good. Realistically, England is the best place for food, because of the choice you get; both to order in and to make for yourself.

The award for the gastronomic shithole of the world goes to Albania. Meals consist mostly of as much meat as possible stuffed onto a plate of potatoes. This meat being of a very dubious quality and origin. There is a big tomato based salad as well. That sounds like a healthy option but any chance of that is destroyed by the addition of endless fistfuls of salt. The only flavour left is that of the chippie[28] at the end of a Friday night.

If Albanians want to go posh, they take the innards out of creatures and then throw the edible parts away. So, at an elegant meal, you find yourself eating the stomach, brains, eyes, and testicles of a goat. There was one occasion when I sat next to my wife eating the salty testicles of another one of God's creatures. Of course, you are trapped by the traditions that heathens inflict on their guests. If you do not eat all of the vile rubbish in front of

---

[28] Fish and Chip Shop: traditional stop on the way home for a well-balanced, nutrioous meal after a night down the pub.

you, then you are insulting them. If you do manage to clean your plate without regurgitating it all back up, then they decide you love it so much that you must have more and more. Eventually, you have to go with the first option and insult everyone. It's the only way to stay alive.

Worst drink? Wait for it: Albania. Most Eastern European countries offer an aniseed-flavoured alcoholic beverage called Raki. In some places, it's called Ouzo, or Sambuca. In Bulgaria, they produce Raki rather in the same way that we treat fine spirits here. They age it for up to 15 years, and casque it in different types of barrels to create different flavours. So you receive all the joys of fine and gentle supping over the long winter months. In Albania, the process is a little different. They place any available fruit and dead creatures in a plastic bottle with lots of sugar. It ferments. It's traditionally drunk at any time of the day, including breakfast.

Every Albanian will tell you that his grandfather from this or that village produces the best Raki. Probably from dead children, or something. But I have yet to notice a significant difference in any that I have tried. Someone did buy an expensive version once but forgot to remove the 'paint stripper' label from the side of the bottle. It was always served in water bottles as camouflage. I was six foot tall with good eyesight and a full head of hair when I went to Albania. I rest my case.

The quality of available drink was one of the reasons that I decided to return to England and settle down with a family, a steady job and a home. Like everyone else. How screwed could one man get?

Chapter Eight: My Return Home - The Court Case

I didn't leave the Foreign Office in a peaceful way. As you are about to see, the whole story is another one of general mayhem and great misfortune. I have never told the tale in full. At least until now.

I think it was May 2007 when I decided to bring my girlfriend over from Albania to the UK to meet my parents in Norfolk. By then, I was divorced (again!), but I had met my girlfriend's family, and that is a serious step towards an engagement in Albania. And, in that country, engagement is really the equivalent of marriage. In fact, the marriage ceremony can be little more than a tea and bun fight, the engagement is the main event.

Who would have believed that this decision would have resulted in well over a million pounds of public money being spent on an investigation that lasted three years? That it would have concluded in a nine-week Crown Court trial in London, with full legal teams headed by QC's?[29] That it would have resulted in 500 lever arch files full of evidence, TV links to Albania, the testimony of around 40 witnesses, the involvement of the bloody Daily Mail, and some six months of research by the

---

[29] Queen's Counsel: high ranking barrister, appointed on the recommendation of the Lord Chancellor of Great Britain. The first Lord Chancellor was Francis Bacon (1561-1626) who was legal advisor to Queen Elizabeth the First.

Metropolitan Police's Serious Crime Squad and the Foreign Office in Albania? That it would have meant me facing the possibility of eight years' incarceration in that rather smelly place where the Crown Jewels are held? All because of a long weekend trip? It seems a bit excessive, even for 'Uber Disaster Man', does it not?

So why on earth did it happen? Because I took my girlfriend along. Yes, that was almost all it was. It is true that I had started an argument with our government over their pathetic visa control methods. This had not made me flavour of the month at the Foreign Office. Remember, I had been a visa officer for some seven years by that point. The place I was posted to was (still is) a dump and everyone wants to leave. The UK has a very weak appeals process when it comes to defending application refusals. So, you need to ensure you make an extremely strong case for refusal in the first place. To achieve this, you must know the country and the local conditions, and you need to complete the paperwork and interview the applicants correctly. Then your colleagues back home will have the option to continue to refuse someone who is, very likely, an illegal immigrant.

But there was a problem with my approach. The British Government had decided it was better to try and reduce the number of refusals, and just accept the paperwork provided. Factories were producing these documents throughout Eastern Europe at the time. It's my opinion that the government had simply decided that it could not afford effective border control and were just going to let it go. A future government could be left to clean up the resulting social mess. So, it was first blood to the Foreign Office. I was a hated man because I was good at my job. Others listened to me, which made it worse. The lamb walked to the slaughter unknowing.

Because I was not engaged to my future wife at the time of the trip in question, my status was only that of a 'boyfriend'. Therefore, a Chaperone was appointed to accompany us. I had previously issued this man with a UK entry visa. I hadn't allowed him the usual six months on it because I was not 100% happy with his application. I had restricted it to one month so that the immigration officers would ask him a few questions when he landed. I'd had no grounds to refuse the request outright. He'd returned to Albania after his UK visit, and there had been no issues. Now, we come to my trip and the two mistakes that I made. If I hadn't, the whole mess might have been avoided.

In a posting where you have more than one Visa Officer, you are not supposed to interview an applicant a second time if you know them personally. However, it's not always practical to avoid this. If you have to do it, then it must be reported. Fair enough. It cuts out fraud.

Obviously, I knew my girlfriend and the Chaperone, so they were interviewed by my colleague. However, the Chaperone had decided to bring his Mistress along on the trip. I didn't say what happened after marriage in Albania, did I? To confuse things, this couple had also made a separate application to visit relatives in London at the same time. When they came in for interview, the applications were split. My colleague interviewed the people that I knew, and I got the Mistress, who I didn't.

This was all correct procedure. My colleague checked the identity of my girlfriend, and that we had an authentic relationship, as she had not been to the UK before. All was fine. I interviewed the Mistress. She had previously been refused a visa and, to begin with I did not realise that she was to be part of my trip home. When the penny dropped, of course, I should have got my colleague to finish the interview. But because the woman would be travelling with me, and within sight the whole time, I just made notes to that effect. I wrote it all down on the application forms. What I should have done was submit it in a separate letter.

We arrived on UK soil at Gatwick Airport. The bloody halfwit immigration officer decided to stop the Chaperone again. While she was asking me about the arrangements, she got it into her head that I had issued him with his current visa, as well as the one a couple of months before. She put in a call to Tirana[30] to check it out. The rot started there.

When we returned to Albania three days later, I took the whole party, and their passports, to see my boss. Just to show him that all was as it was supposed to be. Not one of the people involved ever returned to the UK on the strength of any visa that I wrote. In fact, I had only issued the Mistress a restricted visa because I did not know her, and had some concerns.

The check instigated by the immigration officer led to my suspension from my post. The allegation was that I had given a visa to a friend. Despite the fact that the signature on the visa belonged to my colleague. Despite the fact that she confirmed that she had written it. Despite the fact that nothing untoward had happened on the UK trip. It seemed that a crime had to be found to bugger me up.

By the end of 2007, it was decided that this was grounds to give me the sack. I appealed against this. I met with representatives of the independent appeals committee, and the Foreign Office. I was accompanied by my QC. The Foreign Office were hammered. The law states that it should take three days to get a judgement, but I was confident that I had my job back, and everything would

---

[30] Capital city of Albania.

return to normal. Despite the six months of pain and upset. I wandered over the road to Whitehall for a beer. While I was sat there, a call came through on my mobile. I had lost the appeal. There was no time to register another. I was under arrest for fraud. I swallowed that beer rather quickly.

I turned myself in at Victoria Police Station. Like the dangerous fugitive that I was. I got a lawyer and spent the next few hours listening to a long list of seemingly unrelated questions about my job. This was the first of a series of nice little meetings. They went on for almost three years. At one stage, they even asked me when I first had sex with my girlfriend. To be honest, I never really understood the allegations against me until we got to court.

The accusations centred on my meetings with a foreign businessman in Albania. He was a Recruitment Consultant, who had been seeking permits for locals to work in care homes in the UK. These permits are issued by the Home Office, not the Foreign Office, but obviously, the workers need visas as well. It's not an uncommon situation. I had come across the same set of circumstances in Bulgaria. I'd followed procedure, obtaining permission from my boss to meet with the businessman, and set out a clear agenda with him. from the start. We would check the personal details of each applicant and interview them, as was legally required. As it happened, some of the applicants seemed a little nervous during those interviews, but that is not unusual. Afterwards, my boss even expressed the thought that I had been too strict with them. Some 30 of them were eventually given visas and went to the UK. The prosecution contended that I had accepted money to grant them.

At the trial, all these Carers appeared as witnesses for the prosecution. They all spoke English, and their paperwork relating to their visa applications were all in order. They confirmed that they had been thoroughly checked in Albania and had been fully interviewed. They all confirmed that I had done this work. The Middleman in Albania had even reported to his English counterpart that I had caused delays by doing my job too well. I had met this Middleman three times, once about business. When he was in Tirana, he frequented the same pub that I did with my colleagues. The Deputy Ambassador noted that I did not talk shop with him at all. In fact, this guy was there to watch football on the TV, which I have no interest in at all. There was no money trail because there was no money involved. The judge threw this part of the allegation out.

The foreign businessman, however, was fund guilty of 'Conspiring to use false instruments.' In other words, the court decided that he had used forged paperwork to convince officials in the Home Office that his clients were qualified to take jobs in the UK that could not be filled by British or EU nationals. Hence, they received their work permits. These charges were not related to me.

So, what else was involved? Well, they'd checked all the visas that I granted to applicants with my girlfriend's family name. Her name is as common in Albania as 'Smith' is in England. They checked all the pub owners that had applied, not realising that a pub in Albania can be anything from a hole in the wall to a going concern like a large Irish bar. Why check all these and ask me about them? All the information was there in the documents and the interview records. They were not even familiar with the interview timings that we had to achieve, and the statistical methods that formed the basis of those. The obvious fact that I had one of the highest refusal rates in the entire world may have served to demonstrate that I was not a soft touch.

There were other reports by representatives of the Foreign Office against me. They had examined my phone records and tried to make something of my calls and text messages to and from Albania. It's true that I couldn't prove 100% of these communications were to and from my girlfriend, by then my wife, or calls she had made and received. But the timings and the telephone numbers concerned made it pretty obvious. There were calls to her parents, her sister, her college friends, and so on.

To cut a long story short, the trial lasted nine weeks, which included three days of me on the stand. Witness after witness stated that I had, in fact, done an excellent job as a Visa Officer, with no problems. Witnesses from the Foreign Office were made to look stupid. The result was that I was acquitted by a unanimous jury. I left feeling 100 years older.

My QC advised me that I could take the Foreign Office apart for wrongful dismissal, but I had neither the funds nor the heart for it. The rich and famous do that, not the normal and poor. About six colleagues at the Foreign Office resigned in anger over my treatment, proving that there was honour amongst some of them!

So, in the end, what had all our tax money been spent on? Why had I lost my job and had my photo printed in the Daily Mail? Because I took my wife-to-be on a trip to the UK.

It was not a great start to my return to the UK but, on the bright side, my son, Noel, was born in August 2010. I am so proud of him. It was a pity my mother-in-law moved in with us. To stay forever. It was a pity that my wife took Noel away to Albania for months on end. Her employment record was also a problem. As was her temper. Now we are divorced, and she has agreed to let me see him. Well, the court told her to, and she is already in a spot of bother for attacking me. For once in my life, I occupy the moral high ground!

I think it's time to kick misfortune out. I am sick of being on the bottom of the wart on the arse of the universe. But misfortune and I are still friendly bedfellows, whether I like it or not. As you are about to see.

Chapter Nine: Shitty Health

At the beginning of November 2012, I was suffering from a heavy cold and a sore throat. There was a nasty bug going around. Everyone seemed to have it. I popped into to see my doctor to get something to shift it. I'd also coughed up a little blood, so she sent me straight to the hospital for x-rays. The next day I went back for them to check my throat. The diagnosis followed. I have throat cancer. Of course. How bloody obvious. Why couldn't it just be the cold that everyone else had? Because I am 'Uber Disaster Man.'

Numerous tests began. They included a biopsy on Christmas Eve, ruining my chance for a good Christmas dinner. A tracheotomy is booked for mid-February. So, I face losing the ability to indulge in my favourite pastime: talking shit. Also, several taste buds will be removed, affecting the enjoyment of my other favourite hobby: eating and drinking. Other tests all confirm that my lungs, kidneys, liver, heart, and other vital organs are all in great shape. The cancer just happened. It wasn't because of an unhealthy lifestyle, which would have been easier to accept. Maybe stress caused it. Maybe the Great Being just wants to destroy his toy.

As the weeks passed after the diagnosis, I got sicker. There was a ping-pong ball growing in my neck. By mid-January, I was so ill that I was dragged into hospital. Things improved a lot the first night inside. I was lying there listening to all the moans and screams when the ward was suddenly filled with blokes in prison guard uniforms. They were chained to some hobbit with a bloody nose. Our oldest resident, Albert, was not affected by the uproar. He just continued getting out of bed and wandering around in the nude.

The following day, further tests revealed another diagnosis: diabetes. Nothing more has been said about that since, so I'm just going to shut up about it. But it did mean I got to do a 12-hour starvation diet, which was fun. My escape plans came to nothing, so I stayed on the ward for another night. The prisoner was removed around dawn. A chorus of gunshots and it was all over. In his place came a pilot with skin cancer. He was a nice bloke and the same age as me.

The original occupant of the bed opposite mine had vanished, and been replaced by a traffic policeman who had been admitted because of a constant nosebleed. But he experienced a greater problem that night. The fair, 82-year old, stripping Albert went walkabout again and tried to get into his bed. There was so much leg-pulling the following day that the policeman's other nostril starting bleeding and he ended up with two tampons stuck up his nose. It meant another night on the ward for him, which he found disgusting, but the pilot and I found very amusing. By the look on her face, his wife was rather confused by the whole thing. I was paroled shortly afterward.

Eventually, the great day of the operation arrived. I was back in the hospital on the Coltishall Ward, saying hi to the nurses again. At least, they are interesting people to be around. Patients who have tracheotomies aren't much of a rival in the conversational stakes. You're hardly likely to have a long chat with them.

I went into surgery at 8.00 a.m. on 13" February 2013. It was supposed to be a 12-hour operation to remove the growth. The idea was to take my throat out and replace the feeding tube with a part of my leg. I awoke a little after six hours. I was unable to speak, as I'd expected. I wrote out a joke for the nurse; my first words without a voice: "Am I dead? Is this heaven? Where are the virgins?" It fell flat. It dawned on me that something had gone wrong. The surgeon arrived and explained that the cancer had grown too quickly, and it was in too risky an area for the operation to be completed. I was still wasted and out of my tree on the drugs. All I knew was that my right leg hurt, and l still had a bloody hole in my neck and ten tubes coming out of my body.

My family came to visit around 9.30 pm, trying to locate the wasteland that was their son and brother. I think the phrase 'Roadkill' is a pretty accurate description of how I must have looked. I bore a close resemblance to a squirrel that has been hit by a Heavy Goods Vehicle. At speed. Come to think of it, I would make a hefty bet that I was feeling just about the same as that unlucky animal.

So, what happens now? Well, I have to be repaired from the results of the operation first. A partial tracheotomy is required to assist with the chemotherapy I must have. Possibly in 3 weeks' time. One week in the hospital for that, followed by two weeks recovery. Then one week in the hospital again, and another fortnight recovering at home. The same again with the follow-up radiology. Then a check to see if the growth has shrunk sufficiently to allow the full operation to take place. Nothing is certain. So, I will carry on writing this section; at least until I can get out of the hospital and back home.

It's now six days after my operation. When I write a concerto about it, I'm going to call it 'The Raping of My Organs.' Currently, I have a diet of liquid food that goes straight into my stomach, via a tube stuck up my nose. I have a plastic stick in my throat, and I cough up phlegm on a regular basis and dribble down my chest all the time.

My weak right leg is numb and not fully operational. A couple of years back, I had 18 months of extreme pain trying to walk with a stick because of this leg. I spent a couple of hundred pounds on osteopath bills at least. In the end, a piece of it was not required to rebuild me. Maybe it will never be needed.

I have only one pump in me now to help with my breathing, but I still cannot speak a word. This is becoming a real nuisance as I recover, and need to ask for things. I want to eat real food again, but I can't. Neither of these issues is likely to be resolved for some time.

I may get out of this hospital in a weeks' time, provided the pain has reduced. When that happens, I assume I will be left with the pain caused by the cancer, which is a mild annoyance compared to the pain of the cure. Then, hopefully, I will regain a little speech, and there will be at least some limited eating options. Not great, but, at least, I will be at home.

Of course, a long stay in hospital does not often lend itself to a pleasantly humorous time. In fact, surprisingly enough, a cancer ward is often not the funniest place to be. But here is where the Almighty's plan for me begins to make sense. In fact, he has played a blinder by making me Mr. Cock-Up. All the strange episodes in my life have been preparing me for this one thing: to see the funny side of cancer.

Chapter Ten: Daily Life on a Cancer Ward

The worst sign to get stuck on your door in a hospital is 'Nil by Mouth'. I can live with this sign appearing in my many marriage contracts but when it relates to the loss of food, including Sunday roasts, then this is a tragedy the like of which has not been seen since the events of September 1st, 1939 on the Polish/German border. So now I spend my days with sawdust sludge going up my nose. I now dream of real food. On the bright side, I have no sense of smell so I have to see food before it makes me hungry, and I can fart in a lift and care not. However, once you are well enough to get moved to a soft diet, then your first meal of tomato soup, jelly and ice cream makes the best Christmas dinner you can recall seem like a McDonald's happy meal after ten pints of a very inferior lager.

One swift point to all of you interested in nasal feeding! While you do not feel anything at all, the stupid thing can fall out of your stomach. We had a scare on one night when the plasters sticking it on to my nose started to undo and I found myself stuffing my own pipe back inside me! The doctor then had to try to get me to explain exactly what I did and why I was writing while choking at four in the morning. She tried sticking a metal wire down the pipe but this didn't seem to help. In the end, she decided that the tests of acidity of the fluid in the pipe were sufficient to prove that it was still in my stomach. She guessed and hoped for the best. Well, she was right. I had no idea at the time that there were many hi-jinks and jolly japes with tubes and wires in my immediate future. But more on those later.

Hospital Radio is a wonderful institution. The DJ came around and asked for my requests. I chose 'Silence is Golden' by the Tremeloes and 'The Sound of Silence' sung by a Welsh male voice choir. My sense of humour was praised on the radio. 'And here's a couple of requests by Mark Griffith on Coltishall ward. He is a tracheotomy patient with a fabulous sense of humour. The only man here to ask for songs of silence when he has no voice!' I was asked for another request a couple of days. The dedication for this one went: '…and I met Mark from Coltishall ward again, and this time, he wishes to make a dedication in honour of all those patients at the N and N[31] with the no oral feeding sign on their door. Here is 'Food Glorious Food' from the musical 'Oliver!' If the DJ visits again, I will go for 'Always Look on the Bright Side of Life' from 'Monty Python's Life of Brian'.

My recovery from the operation goes up and down, of course. As I've said already, I was 'road kill' on a drug induced high the day after the procedure. There was slow improvement afterwards until they attempted to

---

[31] The Norfolk and Norwich Univeristy Hospital.

connect my lungs to the voice box, which I still have at present. I almost drowned in my own dribble and spent all day coughing up mucus and blood. It was jolly painful. I recovered from that, but I was still silent and unable to eat.

Immediately after the operation my neck was the size of my head. I looked like a Russian mafia man! My head was attached to my body by a mass of metal staples and cotton. There was one large hole in my neck with an inch of plastic tube hanging out through which to breathe. Or, in reality, cough. From this hole and the edges of it, I continually dribbled thick mucus and blood. For some reason, this was also coming out of a hole in my shoulder. I was hooked up to four pumps, a drip for feed in my nose, and a cannula in my hand. This last tube allowed the easy flow of one of the ten drugs I was on. For good measure, my right leg was also paralysed, and I could not turn my head at all. In fact, I could barely move at all. A thick bed of mucus was entwined with the hair on my chest. My pyjama bottoms didn't fit so my testicles and penis just hung out to one side, made worse by the fact that I was attached to a urine bag. As a final, crowning touch, I was wearing a huge pair of bright yellow Homer Simpson slippers. There were two advantages I had at that stage. Firstly, I had no sense of smell so I did not know how badly I stank. Secondly, I was totally stoned on morphine.

14 nights after I entered that little holiday camp for the mentally concerned, I still could not speak or eat. But I was regaining control of the dribbling and getting some feeling back in my lower regions. I had no pumps or wires in me apart from the feeding tube in my nose and the breathing tube in my neck. The metal staples were gone (I never want to see a staple remover again), and while the leg remains dead, it's viable to walk again. The pain in my leg was actually preferable to the pain before the operation. Not a bad swap. My neck was still very fat like a podgy aristocrat in a satirical cartoon, but I looked more like a rabid Santa Claus really. This is because I cannot shave. Areas of my face are normal, but others are badly bruised and some are still paralysed. So a shave would be complicated. It would be nice to think that the cancer has been numbed out of existence but, as the drugs wear off, I can feel it reasserting itself. Never mind. In a couple of weeks, the cancer and I could have a lovely punch up; one on one.

I was moved from the Coltishall ward to Gissing Ward. Two other people were having the operation done and they needed the bed space. I was in recovery so I could be looked after on another ward that did not specialise in tracheotomies. Or perhaps they just got fed up with me and threw me out. Ungrateful fools. I was the one that bought the Valentine's card for all the nurses there. Ok, one card amongst 24 women is not great. Not that they knew it was me, of course. Whatever the reason, I was transferred.

As a patient, alarm bells start going off when you are wheeled down an ever-darkening corridor that leads up to a barbed wire fence and a massive wooden door. Above the door is emblazoned the motto 'Sanari aut Mori': 'To be Cured or to Die'. Coltishall was a specialist ward and I was looked after in the intensive care section. Gissing (aka 'Guessing') is a general ward, with some staff who allegedly have knowledge of people with breathing problems. I realised at once that the level of health care had changed. Small clues gave it away. The Trade Union poster claiming that Florence Nightingale's so-called modernisation of the health care service was undermining jobs. The large number of druids and leeches was also a worry.

But I did get my own room. It took a while for them to pull out most of the brushes and mops but it suited me. I can't sleep lying down anyway. I convinced myself that it was an upgrade rather than solitary confinement after a failed escape attempt. There was a view of the main atrium and I had my own toilet/washroom. Leaving the curtains and the door to the washroom open at the same time when I performed my ablutions got some amazing looks from the general public. And probably some letter of protest.

I could not sleep at night so instead, I sat up, listening to the cries of the weak and wounded around the ward. They called out for water, for their mothers, or just for someone to end it all. I soon realised why. On Coltishall Ward, you pressed your emergency button and someone was there within a minute or two. Depending on what you needed, your request was dealt with in an average time of about ten minutes. The same was not true on Guessing Ward. It was half an hour before anyone turned up, and your request might get completed in the next seven hours. It took that long for one dose of tablets that I needed.

In a sense, I am fortunate because, as a partial tracheotomy patient, they have no idea what to do for me. So I get left alone a bit. However, they have to help me with some things. The feeding tube in my nose fell out. When that happened, they did not check if it had come out of my stomach or not, the nurse just pulled the whole thing out. Originally, I'd had it fitted when under anaesthetic because I have a very badly bruised throat and a great bloody cancer growing there. It's damn difficult to get anything past that lot without a hell of a lot of pain. To resolve the problem, the staff on Guessing Ward just ignored it. For a couple of days. The only sustenance I had for that time was sugar water going through a cannula. All of my tablets were forgotten, apart from the ones to control my epilepsy. They got those into me by ramming them up my bottom. I was not amused.

Finally, on day three, the cavalry arrived in the form of a surgeon and a doctor from my medical team. A camera and light on a probe were guided up one nostril, and then down, to guide the feeding tube back into my stomach. It finally reached its destination, accompanied by a lot of discomfort. All that was left to do was for someone to make the official check that the tube was in the stomach and connect me back to my feed, and my medication. I was starving by then. Well, they worked as fast as they possibly could. Four hours later, some total drip masquerading as a nurse shuffled into my room. She grabbed the tube and pulled the stabilising wire out from the centre of it. Now, this is the wire that's used to x-ray the feeding tube. To confirm it is in the stomach. It only takes seconds. Why did she do it? 'Just to show you how confident I am that this is in the right place'.

But there was a slight problem. She still had to prove it. If the end of the tube is not in the stomach, sawdust sludge would have gone rushing randomly through my internal organs. I would have suffered all forms of hell. Her alternative method was to draw some fluid up through the tube. If the ph of the fluid was acid, then the tube was in the stomach. Fine. But there's another slight problem: I hadn't eaten for two days so there was no fluid to test. She left. That was her solution; she just left.

I got another nurse and, three hours later, it was confirmed that everything was ok, and feed and drugs could go where they should. At times like that, it was a blessing that I was mute.

That same drippy nurse had to give me an injection now and then. She was the only one who held the needle like a dart and just thumped it in. She was like some cartoon representation of a nurse. Sadly, she was real and, even worse; she was looking after me. But she did manage to clean my room up of discarded medical equipment. I'm not sure how many people she told that she had done this taxing, five-minute job but I guess doing her week's work in one go was probably worthy of comment. There was even a health care worker who communicated with me by shouting. Very slowly. Based on the fact that I could not speak. I know what a Frenchman must feel like now.

Obviously, someone from my medical care team had a word about the standard (and dangerous) health care available on the Guessing Ward. All of a sudden, my visiting family were subjected to a lot of pathetic excuses, and comments from the nurse such as "you know me, I would never let you down"; "always around for you"; "we get on really well". Etc, etc. No, not true; you are a totally dangerous dickhead. Please leave me alone.

Although I wouldn't have thought it possible, the quality of patient seems to be lower as well. I'd assumed that illness made no allowances for class, employment, size of bank account or educational history. But I met one patient wandering around Guessing Ward trying to bum drugs because he was getting withdrawal symptoms. I tried to explain to him that he should not worry. He was just clean and sober, and this is what the real world is like. Of course, I ended up following him around, hoping for the dog ends of any drugs that he might find. After the awful realisation that what I'd told him was completely true.

Then there are the relatives to consider. Because there will be a happy day when you'll be released. To taste that sweet joy of freedom; to have more than a six foot square space to live in, to be able to sleep and wake without fear. To able to stop worrying about your trousers falling down, potentially lethal injections or some arsehole taking your blood pressure, temperature, pulse, and oxygen in blood percentage. Every four hours.

Of course, I am only assuming what this day must feel like as it hasn't happened to me yet. My horizon is looking a little blank at this point. But I can assume it is like winning the lottery or being demobilised from the army after surviving active service throughout the First World War. You're a little scared but overjoyed that you made it. Then your bloody relatives refuse to take you back because they've forgotten who you are. A thought suddenly dawns on you: 'you mean I'm still married?' That is what it feels like. Do not pass go. Do not collect £200.[32] What happens to me now I don't know, and I'm scared to ask. Just how near is the crematorium to the ward? Is this where the spare human organs come from? I am going to be so nice to my mummy and daddy and Karen and Chris from now on. Please do not leave me on the Guessing Ward.

I was very proud of myself the other day, having earned the official title of a 'complex patient'. Unfortunately, this has nothing to do with any philosophical bent that I may have; it just means that I have a whole load of things that have fallen off me at the same time. As a result, many different departments are involved in my care and a whole team of people are working in unison to put Humpty Dumpty together again. The list, as I know it, is as follows:

1. One surgeon in charge of the physical removal of cancerous growth
2. Plastic surgeons to rebuild my oesophagus
3. The Anaesthetists
4. The Tracheotomy Team

---

[32] The rules in the popular board 'Monopoly'; usually enforced when you are sent to jail.

5. The Speech Therapists
6. Dietician
7. Physiotherapists (Body)
8. Physiotherapists (Breathing)
9. A stomach consultant, and assistants, for current feeding arrangements and gastrostomy
10. One head of Chemotherapy and Radiology
11. Chemotherapy team
12. Radiology team
13. Pain relief team
14. Pharmacy
15. Registrar
16. Ear Nose and Throat doctors
17. Ear Nose and Throat nurses and full support team
18. Local GP
19. District nurses

Of course there are many others involved with the various x-rays, laboratory tests and numerous and varied pre-assessments that were required.

I am very glad that we have all kept our NI[33] payments

---

[33] National Insurance: a system of contributions paid by workers and employers in the UK towards the cost of certain state benefits, such as free medical care under the NHS.

up to date! It wasn't until just now that I have realised how many people are involved in this project. So, if any of you are feeling sorry for me because it can be boring in hospital please fear not! In any one day, I will be having meetings and tests with at least some of these people. Nearly all of them are a delight. Mind you, all the nurses on Guessing ward are convinced that my 75-year-old mother is my wife and that my sister is my daughter. That makes me feel just great. Ego kicked right into touch.

The 26th of February, 2013 was a red letter day. My first real meal in more than two weeks. But matters involving your health can change very quickly. The great power had allowed me to think that I was getting better. I was almost ready to go home and prepare for my course of Chemotherapy. But it had another unpleasant surprise in store. After the meal, the doctors came in to change my tracheotomy tube for a new one. This would have allowed for more eating and the possibility of speech. But they discovered that I was still losing some of my food, or dribble, into my lungs. That can cause infection so my release was cancelled. I could be stuck here for another week at least, and I'm back to 'Nil by Mouth'.

There is a chance that Thursday's review will allow me home earlier. But I do not hold out much hope. I am sad. For most people such a knock back would be a dreadful worry, of course, but worse was to come for me. My feeding pipe fell out. It would not go back in without choking me. As a result, I have had nothing to eat or drink, and no pain relief. There is only one orifice left that allows my epilepsy tablets to enter my system – that of my cute little bottom! It's a very interesting way to get to know your nurse, but it does not work. I have had two partial seizures. Given the extent of my problems, I decide that I do not want neurology specialists added to my team. So we'll just forget it. Let the professionals concentrate on getting that feeding tube around the cancer. Then I can carry on as 'normal'.

Shortly after this latest setback, I was allowed to go home for the weekend. For the next few months, this became the pattern of my life; resting at home between visits to the hospital for chemotherapy.

Chapter Eleven: Batty Betty & other characters encountered on the great exploding stomach expedition

06/07/13 to 24/07/13: Mulbarton Ward

Tale of a Toilet

I am sat in a chair outside my current home: Bed 3, Bay 7, Mulbarton Ward, Norfolk & Norwich Hospital. I am gazing out of the window at my metre square of sky, and the rear end of the canteen and the portacabins, supplied courtesy of Carters, the builders. It's a pleasant day, but it's about to be interrupted by the latest achievement in nursing, courtesy of Batty Betty.

It all started with one almighty thump emanating from the toilet opposite our bay, followed by a weak, frail voice squawking 'Oh, F**k!' Imagine for a moment that you are the sweet little old lady involved in this mishap. You have cancer. You are receiving Chemotherapy. You feel absolutely terrible and you are being sick all the time. Now, you've wet yourself and fallen over inside the toilet. You can't move, and you're locked in. Could life get any worse than that? Well, yes, it could. Batty Betty cries out; "You no worry, I come help." I gave up all hope for her right then. The old lady probably started to weep.

I have to admit that Batty Betty does have a heart of gold. She is good with getting cannulas into deep veins after all other potential entry points have closed up. But otherwise, her talent lays only in her desperate attempts to help but cause chaos instead. In hindsight, I can say that she proved to be a great source of much-needed humour. With a lot of hindsight.

Back to the current crisis. A frail, elderly cancer patient has fallen over in a confined space and cannot move. Now, toilet doors on a hospital ward do not lock as such. They are designed to be very easy to open for just such a circumstance as this. If the door handle is lifted and turned in the opposite direction, it overrides the lock and the door opens outwards into the corridor. This prevents any risk of harm to the patient if they have fallen against the door, and gives the nurse easy access. It's very simple and effective. Betty, on the other hand, is very simple and ineffective. She finds an unknown source of strength from somewhere deep within, and smashes the door inwards, crashing into the sick woman on the floor. By now, she's already making her peace with God, because she's fully aware of who is spearheading her rescue bid. Luckily for her, the Ward Sister intervenes, explaining a few facts to Bat while other nurses pull the old woman from the wreckage.

Batty's M.O. in a nutshell: an honest effort to help that finishes in disastrous failure and chaos. The next exam-

ple occurred merely a few hours after the lavatorial rescue attempt.

My Batty Wash and Change

One of the pleasures I get out of being pathetically sick
is having someone help to wash and change me. It's not
humiliating at all. My favoured assistant is big Karl. He
can tidy up, wash and change me, and redo my bed perfectly in a few moments. Given my requirements, it's no
mean feat to manage all this efficiently. And it's very
important. Karl is a health assistant, not a nurse, so does
not deal with drugs, or other medications and he is out-
ranked by everyone, apart from the guy who cleans the
toilets.

On the day in question, Karl had just started to clean up
my living area, before sorting me out. Suddenly, Batty
Betty appeared around the curtain to 'help'. Because I
am still mute, I cannot tell her to sod off. I am trapped.
In the hospital hierarchy, she is in charge of Karl so he
cannot object either. Her first act of assistance is to
knock over all the inner tubes for my tracheotomy. The
brushes go the same way so she throws them all out,
thus making cleaning the inner tubes impossible. Not
content with such minor calamities, she bounces over to
where Karl is setting up the wash kit on my side table.
She decides to help by making more space and knocks

my orange squash over. So a quick and easy job for Karl has turned into a significant task because he has to wash the bloody floor.

Now the finale! Batty decides to change my pyjama top. This requires switching off the four main lines which connect me to a battery of pumps. These look after my feed, hydration, antibiotics and combined painkillers and anti-sickness drugs. There was a mass of lines, pipes, electrical leads, pumps, nebuliser, extractor, oxygen and even a computer. How do you think she did? My diet ended up as pure morphine, which was useful in one sense as my official pain relief had been disconnected and utterly lost. That wire took ages to retrace. I believe it was finally found attempting to recharge my mobile. I reckon it took Karl about an hour to extract me from the mains! So my morning ended on a cloud of morphine. I became a small bright purple banana!

The Discovery of Magic Spray, or how Betty the Bat tried to sacrifice me!

Now, as promised by the title of this chapter, let's go back a little to how I ended up in here again. Let's talk about my exploding stomach. It was a bit of a mess. Blood and internal fluids were still gushing out of me on day three so I was rushed back into the hospital. It was a reaction to all the steroids they had been pumping into me.

The big issue was to staunch the flow of fluid so repair work could begin. I was still throwing up blood, and every time I moved there was the great risk of more fluid coming out. How on god's sweet earth, my stomach could have retained so much muck I will never know, but by the time I got into hospital it was mostly blood. As I sat there in bed holding my stomach, I looked for the entire world like a Vietnam veteran, or the hero of some anti-war film like Cat in 'All Quiet on the Western Front'. I was in constant agony and was as weak as the intellect of an Albanian. Obviously, no feed could go in and every available vein was taking blood transfusions, water and salts, pain relief and antibiotics. A lot of the cannulas were in painful places, and there was an almost constant struggle to balance the drugs to help with my epilepsy, which was threatening to run amok. Aside from that, all my bodily functions had to be constantly monitored and the wound controlled. So I was a high priority for those first few days. All the medical skill of a specialised ward was put into practice to help me.

Night in a hospital can be terrifying. The early hours is the time when we always feel most alone. But there are worse things than loneliness. Such as sensing the curtain around your hospital bed moving ever so slightly. Such as seeing the demonic features of Batty Betty amidst all the carnage, chaos, blood and pain. With a sinking feeling similar to the captain of the Lusitania, I realised that I was to be her sacrificial victim or 'specialist patient.' Mentally, I prepared myself for the madness to be unleashed upon me, muttering my personal motto: 'Quid est quod me semper?' Why is it always me?

The senior oncology consultant Doctor Roques had left that evening with the following simple instruction. 'Do not do anything with this patient until tomorrow, just keep the bandages as we have them.' With these words of wisdom still ringing in her head, the Bat pulls all the bandages off. What she thought was going to happen I have no idea. She emitted a strange squeak as a massive mess bloody mess began to form. It was rather similar to the breaching of the Ruhr valley dams when they made the acquaintance of a few bouncing bombs.

She just stood staring at my stomach like the full cast of 'Watership Down'[34] looking into car headlights. Then there was the usual sudden burst of energy and enthusiasm. She grabbed all the paper towels out of the dispenser and neatly folded them onto my stomach. It was not a brilliant plan. It did nothing other than turn white paper into red as I continued to bleed. The sponges and gauze that had previously worked in retaining my stomach contents remained in a heap next to me. I inwardly

---

[34] A popular novel, and film, about the adventures of a group of rabbits.

wept as I saw no logical plan in any of her actions. But she had one last trick up her sleeve. It was her Ardennes offensive of 1944, her last bold and desperate bid to save everything. And the humiliation of having to answer the question: 'Why did you screw up his bandages?'

She pierced a plastic bag and hung it on the side of the rig. Next, she glued it to my stomach, or what remained of my chest hair, to be precise. The fluids would now enter the bag. The basic idea was sound, but the Bat's design skills were a little lacking. There were two holes in the bag, and they were in the wrong place.

Modern methods of teaching mean that should a student miss a lesson, then they don't have to worry about it. No need to catch up; the subject you missed simply does not exist. This works for everyone. The child feels no defeat or the pain of thinking that they are stupid. The Bat obviously went to the local chip shop the day Newton's laws were taught so they did not exist for her. Having a bag with an exit hole at a lower point than the entryway caused her no pain. It caused me a shed load of pain, though. The fluids went wild and even tried to go back into the original opening. The Bat could not understand why her plan had failed. She'd thrown in her lot with the crazy glued bag on the belly solution and lost. She'd come up against gravity and finished second.

It was her final card. After it failed, she simply legged it, leaving it to the day shift to resolve the whole debacle. She also managed to leave me with no access to communications, just the button that controls the bed. With all the blood and plastic and paper towels, I must have resembled a grenade attack in a chicken factory. To try and get attention from behind my curtains, all I could do was push the button and go up and down in my bed. The day nurse started her shift by pulling back my curtain to find her patient hanging onto a plastic bag and manically pressing the bed control. Eerily rising and descending like some blood soaked sacrifice to an Aztec god.

The clean up was a long process. Involving a lot of pain with my glued hair. But I found out that there are skin nurses who deal with such issues. They have a magic spray that makes all the glue just give up its stickiness. The plastic bag was easily removed. I am now hooked on this magic spray.

The Bat was absent from the bay where I live for some time after this stunt, but not from the ward. She carries the potential to cause a catastrophe with her like an unexploded time bomb. And she was not finished with me yet.

How to Wake Up Batty Betty Style

After such a miserable time I was overjoyed to be left alone. Later in the week, I had a real good nights sleep, one of the best since before the cancer. I was dreaming of my equivalent of heaven where I had all my toy soldiers with me and I was sorting through them. Then a bloody tidal wave hits. I wake up face to face with the Bat! She makes her normal babbling and cackling sounds and turns like a demented scientist to the grand selection of drips, pumps and pinging machines connected to me in various places. One tube is already swinging wildly around me, spraying out cold, watery, porridge. Most of it has already discharged all down my left-hand side.

I alert the Bat by directing a squirt of this cold fluid in her direction. She explains this latest debacle as follows: 'Ok, ok, I know. It all ok. I tie on next. It ok. I will do in just a moment. Oh dear, Mr. Mark want to pinch Betty? She been bad?' No, Mr. Mark does not want to bloody pinch you, dropkick into next week maybe, but I do want the porridge fountain to stop.

Bat took her usual course of action; stare wide-eyed at the problem. In this case, a quickly spreading porridge puddle in which I was beginning to float. Then she muttered some incantation or other and fitted the tube back into the line. Then off she rattled out of the bay, bashing into any object or person in sight that could result in minor chaos.

Almost immediately afterwards, another nurse arrived. It's possible they are following her. Perhaps they consider her as a possible 5th columnist from the Guessing Ward. It was just as well. This angel of mercy pulled back the curtains to find her patient debating whether to build a dinghy or use the backstroke to move around in his bed. Again I got another hosing down and a full change to start the day. Well, it was that or have Goldilocks and three bears let loose on me.

The final little sting in this little tale of a disastrous wake-up call was that the Bat had used super powers to tie the feeding tube to me. The nurses almost had to resort to getting advice from the builders outside my window to free me from it. I sleep with one eye open now.

Lavatorial Problems

Not every adventure in hospital involved Betty the Bat. I am quite able to cause disaster all by myself. The 15th of July was a fine example of my home-grown stupidity. At 5:30a.m. I was busy making an idiot of myself. Old habits die hard!

I went to the toilet using the urine bottle. It was my fifth one of the night, in fact. Unfortunately, I fell asleep afterwards with my pee distributor still out and in the bottle. I slept without a problem until a few hours later, when I had another lavatorial experience. I can confirm that Archimedes is correct. He displaced bath water. I used urine. My theorem proves that 600ml of urine does not fit into a 500ml container!

The morning shift nurse arrived to find five full urine bottles on my side table and half of one in my bed. Without an accompanying bottle. At least I managed to get washed and changed first that day! In addition, I created a small test. The nurses can use it to train patients in the use of technical equipment, like a urine bottle.

The exam is as follows:

As a patient, you have successfully urinated in the bottle. Do you -

    a)   Pass the bottle to the nurse.

    OR

    b) Continue to use the bottle until you soak yourself in your own pee?

Chapter Twelve: Those Accursed Physiotherapists

I appreciate I need exercise to monitor my breathing, improve my strength and 'buld me up' generally, but I swear these physiotherapists are the Greek equivalent of the Waffen SS Das Reich Panzer Division.[35] However, I am determined I will not swear an eternal oath of allegiance to Beelzebub, the Flaming Angel of Death, or anything else they have in mind.

The usual procedure is that the Physio Officer stands to one side of the treadmill, and barks orders at me to set the pace. The other is behind me, pushing the metal pole with all the pumps on. This pinches at your ankles if you don't move quick enough. This goes on for 20 to 30 minutes a day. I march in fear as far as I dare.

But the first session had its moments. These hard-assed stormtroopers forgot that I am a tracheotomy patient, or a 'trachy' as we are usually called. So when they got me back to bed after all that marching, I started to cough. It turned into an almighty choking fit. There was mucus all over the place. Well, the tough as nails Physio Officers simply fell apart. They ran around terrified, handing me anything within reach in a vague hope of providing assistance. The Zimmer frame, in particular, plumbed

---

[35] A notorious tank division of the Nazi SS that operated during World War II.

the pits of stupidity and outright panic. They no longer stick around after the route march!

Good Morning Mr. Griffith

How do you usually wake up in the morning I wonder? A hug from a partner or a nuzzle from a pet? A nice cup of tea or a screaming alarm clock? I usually wake up around 07:15 a.m. to a very faint aroma of noodles. Given that I have no sense of smell anymore, this is mighty clever! I open my eyes slowly to welcome in another day but instead find myself staring directly into the milk bottle bottomed glasses and the huge staring eyes of Yington Ruddyrud, the blood collector. He lunges forward with his bayonet needle and hits exactly the same spot on my arm that he always does. He collects his six syringes full of my B+ with ruthless efficiency. I remember where I saw his father. He was the model for Hitoshito, the evilest Japanese POW camp commandant in the 'Battle for Boys' comic book I read each week as a youngster.

It is a terrifying way to greet the morning until one recalls that I used to wake up next to my ex-wife. Given how thoughtless she was, it was a miracle that when the mother-in-law came to stay, I wasn't thrown out of bed to sleep on the couch while she took my place. That was when mother in law moved into our one bedroom flat for a two week holiday. Which was slightly extended to two years.

Life with Urine Bottles (again)

My most memorable experience with urine bottles was a couple of weeks ago on a Saturday. I had been urinating a lot, and the results were bright green and contained blood. I was rushed back into the hospital; no detours, straight to Emergency, with my Mum in close attendance.

You have the picture. I am sat up in bed, with my clothes covered in mess and looking like an extra from 'Alien'. The bed sheets are turning red and brown. Fortunately, I no longer have a sense of smell so I was unaware of the stench. The Ward Sister rushed into the carnage with her sleeves rolled up to assist her two nurses. The first thing she did was to get a urine bottle for me, as once again I was desperate to pee. I correctly docked my equipment with the hole of the bottle. It came out and flowed like high tide at Hunstanton[36]. Sadly for me, the Ward Sister is a pillock. She had provided me with a urine bottle with no base. I succeeded in covering myself, and my bed, in my own urine.

---

[36] A popular seaside resort on the North West Coast of Norfolk.

The curtains were pulled back to reveal me holding the two hole bottle, looking seriously annoyed. Literally, pissed off. The result was that my Mum burst into laughter, followed by two nurses and the Trachy specialist. The Ward Sister had vanished by this point. Perhaps it was a test to see how her staff would deal with an escalating emergency. Laugh at it, it seems! I was not amused for the longest time.

Chapter Thirteen: Donut Man

Donut Man is a charming, very helpful person but a little slow to understand my needs probably because I cannot speak. He is so named for two reasons. Firstly, because he is as useful to nursing as a doughnut. Secondly, because you watch him work and say 'doh!' Sure, a touch of of onomatopoeic licence, but I think it's allowed. Karen and I watched him clean one of my inner tubes. You'd take probably three or four minutes. Even without training. Donut Man takes fifteen to twenty. First come the gloves, then the front cover for his clothes. Then he picks up the pot and the dirty and clean canula. He takes everything to the sink. He takes out one dirty one and disposes of it. He comes back with a clean one, then returns to the sink to dispose of another dirty one. Then he comes back with a clean one, returning to the sink to dispose of another dirty one. And so on. Then he picks up a packet of brushes, goes back to the sink, takes out one and brings it over. Then it's back to the sink for another. One at a time. And so it went on! Another moment of hilarity in the hospice!

His colleague I call Sweet but Stupid. My worrying introduction to her was when she arrived to tidy my bed and sort my sheets out. I watched in horrified amazement as each item was taken off my bed one at a time. The same procedure was followed with the contents of my bowl. Then she just put everything back where it had been. Item by item. At the end of this process she asked me if she was a good cleaner. Assuming irony to be beyond (way, way beyond) the conversation, I wrote down that 'I was indebted to her.' Out came a little book, and she wrote it down as well. She asked me what it meant. Great news! She has just begun to learn English. I'm guessing, but I think she may be from the Philippines.

These are the two nursing assistants assigned to me here. Well, all companies have idiots obviously; but I had got both of them. And on the night shift, which made it worse. My full-time home carer, Nick, is also a nursing assistant, but he knows his job inside out. What a contrast.

Another day I asked Sweet but Stupid for the pink sponges from the drawer of the bedside cabinet. When she finally found the drawer, she showed me white brushes. No, it's good but it's not right. Then she finds wipes in a pink packet. But I don't want them, do I? Now Sweet but Stupid is rather lost. I want pink sponges, and I know they are in there because I saw her put them there earlier in the day. But all she sees is the white brushes and a packet with the colour pink on it. She just kept showing the packets to me one at a time for maybe 10 minutes. I have no idea if she thought they would morph into the pink sponges or what! Eventually, she saw the sponges and got them for me!

The final example of calamity features both of these characters. I asked Sweet but Stupid to plug my phone charger in at the hospital. I had the charger in my hand, and there was a spare socket just above me. She did not look at these, but said 'I get nurse'. She came, pointed at the two items and left muttering something that sounded like "Barcelona"![37] My feed tube is in the general vicinity of the socket in question and Sweet but Stupid's first attempt nearly disembowelled me. She tried to turn me inside out 36 times before she had the bright idea of getting Donut Man involved. The sight of them wrestling with the task of putting a plug in a socket with my feeding tube in the way will haunt me for ages. I gave up hope after a short while and just hung onto my feeding tube for grim death. Well, they managed it in the end, but put a knot in the tube that Houdini would be proud of!

One night was peaceful as Donut Man had fufilled his quota of slow/stop mayhem in the morning instead. All he had to do was get my equipment ready after I washed. We had an hour. It took him half an hour to work out how to use a flannel, and the ambulance turned up half-an-hour early. I had finished changing by then, but Donut was under pressure to collect the few items

---

[37] A reference to popular British TV sitcom 'Fawlty Towers.' When waiter Manuel caused another disaster, the excuse given was that he was 'from Barcelona.'

that needed to go with me. The ambulance crew and the rest of us just watched this car crash of an event unfold.

He kept looking at the emergency box, but wouldn't pick it up. Eventually, someone gave it to him to put everyone out of their misery. Then he got hold of the extractor. I had written down for him that it needed to go inside its black case. He actually opened the little purple emergency box twice to see if it would fit in there! By now, there was laughter and clapping from the watching audience. It took Donut Man a while to work out the zip mechanism but, lo, the magic case opened. I bet you've already guessed the next bit. How to get the extractor into the box? Well, he just kept bashing away with it the wrong way around like a demented chimpanzee! Somehow, he turned it and voila, it was in! Then he took it out in celebration, but forgot how to put it back in again.

Thank heavens, we had pre-packed the majority of equipment, and I'd already collected my phone, glasses and anything else I might need. There were just the two inner tubes left to bring. They don't come in a sealed container, so we needed a little box or a bag for them. Donut Man arrives with them in a bloody pillow case. He then proceeded to crush this bundle into the extractor box. Fair play to him, he managed it.

So we were now ready to go, except the last laugh was on me. I suddenly start coughing, and need the extractor and an inner tube! That taught me to laugh at other people. There was a lot of groans because time was pressing by then. So Donut Man was placed on more important duties, such as counting all the tea bags to make sure that we had not been swindled. It kept him out of the way. We left for the hospital slightly bemused by it all, but with the comforting knowledge that should our infant children ever be faced with such a task, they would make a better job of it.

Donut Man helped me to bed in the hospital, where I sit up. It's quicker to stay in bed this way than keep transferring to the chair and back again. I wrote out a clear list of ten items for him to help me with, in order. He read down the list, and did one in the middle, then left. I got him back and had to write out the list one item at a time. Yes; write down the first item. Stop. He does it. Then the next item. And so on. Karen can set me up in ten minutes while chatting. He took over an hour!

I saw him help Bedpan Man on the ward today. He's a chap with bowel issues, obviously. Donut was of invaluable help in this instance, as he blundered into the gents, snatched up one sheet of toilet paper, and wandered back to the disaster area. He then repeated the procedure. Exactly. And so on.

A few nights ago I was having a fabulous dream about playing in the sunny, warm garden in Burghley Street[38], but the day became darker, wet and cold. The ground turned to mud, and there was rubbish all around me. Then I saw the wire and the trenches and heard someone shouting. I felt confusion and fear. There was a terrible smell and taste in my mouth. Lord spare me this hell! It was 1915 at Mons, and the Germans had started their gas attacks.[39] I awoke suddenly, and in relief, I drew a big breath. Massive mistake. There was a reason for the nightmare. Bedpan Man had exploded!

No war scene or Foreign Office training could have prepared me for it. The nurses were lined up at the ward entrance two by two, like animals leaving a sinking ark. They crossed themselves and marched toward the blue curtains. When they returned, they no longer looked human! After the disintegrating pots, and their contents were dropped into a nuclear waste canister out of sight, I could hear the showers, tears and one of them saying; "don't worry, blow bubbles".

Of course, despite the decimation of the nursing staff, Bedpan Man was repaired. It was then that I got a peek behind his blue curtain, and saw the scaffolding they use

---

[38] The street in Kettering where the author grew up.

[39] First major action of the British Expeditionary Forces in the First World War.

to hoist him up for emergencies such as that. The only advantage he has that I can see is an almost never-ending supply of toilet paper from the Health and Safety Executive[40]. I just hope for his sake the paper is soft and absorbent; like the HSE itself. I did learn one thing from witnessing this devilish experience,; what a terrible job emptying a bedpan can be. I feel sorry for the guy who deals with me.

Returning to the day that Donut Man made such a fabulous job of getting me ready for my latest hospital visit, it wasn't over yet. I supposed it served me right for laughing at him in the first place. The nurse came in with my meds an hour late and apologised saying there had been problems. Donut Man walked in behind the nurse with an extra dangerous dumb look on his face, mixed with a sad, crestfallen expression. He was the nurse's errand boy for the drug run. He did ask if he could leave the ward to help out somewhere else, but the nurse wouldn't let him. I took my chance and presented my list of eight things that needed to be done to get me ready for sleep. These were written with Donut Man in mind. It ran something like this: Move wine glass[41] to large table. Move wine bottle to large table. Remove jug of water to kitchen. And so on.

---

[40] Non-departmental public body in the United Kingdom responsible for the regulation and enforcement of health, safety and welfare in the workplace.

[41] By this point, Mark was allowed the occasional glass.

135

Donut Man looked up and down the list a couple of times. He picked up the wine glass and looked for a place on the small table to put it back down again. Then, by luck, he saw the huge table by his side. He hunted around the space on the table for a while, and, after a couple of minutes, put the glass down. He then looked at me, smiled, said 'thank you' and walked off!

But the nurse, who was possibly not his best friend at that moment, called him back saying that "Mark needs our help". Well, he managed to complete some of the tasks, but there was a discussion with each one. Why didn't I keep the wine on the small table? Did you mean this jug of water? Well, there is only one available jug of water on the ward. My table is so small that only one jug will fit on it. You are looking at, and touching the jug in question. Yes, that bloody jug!! He managed that at last and did the urine bottle before his wanderlust took over again. He thanked us and left. The nurse quickly completed the rest of his job, while doing my meds. The two of us waited for the inevitable. After about five minutes came a muffled 'No!' from along the ward somewhere, followed by the inevitable return of the dejected Donut Man. He stood by the toilet like some teenager at his first disco, trying to work out how to dance, ask a girl out, and remain cool all at the same time. He was in a sorry state. The nurse saved the day by requesting his help in putting me to bed. It was a minor inconvenience that through it all I had been lying on a big table!

Donut Man is also good at setting out sheets and pillows, and he's a real whiz with the urine bottle exchange. More little moments to brighten up my day!

And on the penultimate day of my latest incarceration, I find jackass number three. 'Nice but Dim' is also from the Philippines. All I asked for was to have a blanket over the bed. She asked me if I was cold and I said that I was. Her next question was 'Do you want me to open it for you?'; No, of course not, I thought you could just dump a piece of folded material at the bottom of the bed and I would imagine warmth. I explained that I was a bit of a traditionalist and that the blanket covering me would be great. So she got the blanket and my peg and shook it out. I squealed like the fifth little piggy running all the way home! To cap it all, she is actually training one of the other students.

There you go – the story so far. There is fun in all things if you look for it.

Chapter Fourteen: Interview For My Carer

A Note from Sheila Griffith:

Mark had to attend the hospital almost daily, and we had a wonderful band of ambulance crews to ferry us backwards and forwards. They were marvellous, but the only problem was the fact that they collected Mark at the unearthly hour of 8 o'clock each morning. Now, both Mark and I are not early risers and to get myself and Mark up, washed and dressed, have all his medication and be ready to face these cheerful souls was quite a feat!

I was getting very tired and realised that once Mark was back home permanently, I would need some help. So we asked for a full-time carer. This is the story of the first interview Mark and I had (don't forget, Mark couldn't speak and had to write everything down!)

We have just had the interview from hell. We have found the Zimbabwean version of Satan. Quite how difficult it was for us to find someone so completely unfitted to care for me remains one of the great mysteries of the modern world. I now plead with the universe not to leave me with this woman. Until the company burns her application, I am at the mercy of the Lord God Almighty again. So what was wrong with her? There follows a brief summary, covering the main points:

1. For a start, she obviously hates me. There was almost zero communication between us. She vaguely spoke in my direction a couple of times. She did not look at me.

2. She has slightly different interests than me. I am fascinated by the political, social and military history of the 1800's and 1900's. I study many scientific topics at an amateur level. I love nature and the wonderful variation of the English countryside, and, as a gregarious person, I enjoy speaking to people of all types. She likes the shopping channel.

3. I was unaware of exactly what language she was speaking, but it was not English. I spent a decade abroad and have been married to women who did not speak my native tongue, and I only managed to work out 50% of her mutterings. Mum had no hope of understanding her at all.

4. The temperature in my house is a steady 24.5 Centigrade (76 Fahrenheit). It was too cold for her. Heaven, help that bill!

5. The lunch she brought with her was a heated sand-wich stuffed with onion. Mum said it stank. I am sure that I saw an empty collar with 'Tiddles' and an address. After three or four months, we'd probably have to fumigate the house.

6. She wants to return to her tribal lands again for the month of December. So she would be absent for a quarter of the time she is required.

7. She was very blunt and possessed not even a flicker of politeness. There was not a trace of the normal social niceties, such as complementing your host on a lovely home.

8. She had absolutely no interest in Norwich. She just told us that Leeds[42] was better and talked about the distance to London.

9. She refuses to walk anywhere, even up the road from the bus stop. When Mum said it was a lovely stroll into the city, she was blunt to the point of rudeness. She does not walk.

---

[42] A city in West Yorkshire in England.

10. She goes to bed at 10 pm. She did indicate that 12 pm would be ok, but it seemed to Mum that the ability to be flexible was not on the table.

11. She does have other interests. Going out and music. We never expanded on that, which I consider a blessing. I suspect she meant going out to a club. I doubt if it would have been a folk club. Or a library. Or a wander in the country for that matter.

12. Her previous experience has been with old people and in a hospital. Well, I suppose by the end of this interview I had aged, and I was considering spending my recovery back in hospital. Batty Betty would have been preferable to this woman.

13. She assumed that all the house and washing was dealt with by a cleaner. I presume she is so wealthy that this is how she deals with her things in Leeds. But in the real world, she would be expected to do this mammoth task for me. Might I suggest that perhaps she is a little lazy by nature?

14. She made many references to an alarm system to alert her during the night if I needed anything. When Mum was out of the room, she quizzed me further, and I explained to her the main concern is the epilepsy. But she pressed me further about having to get up at all. I thought to myself how perfect-

ly reasonable she was about it all. For the paltry sum of say £500 per week, I wouldn't get up twice a night for ten minutes to check if my patient is ok. If I was going to the lavatory or happened to hear him coughing, for instance. So I have decided to die and not make a mess for her. I will go to the bottom of the garden and dig my own grave, jump in and pull the soil over myself. Might I suggest that perhaps she is a little lazy?

15. She mentioned one other hobby; having naps! Well, she'd need them after all her hard work, wouldn't she? Might I suggest she is a little lazy?

16. Given that she refuses to walk a few yards; is concerned by simple house cleaning; has a hobby that involves sleeping and does not wish to check up on me at night, I cannot see her shifting all my equipment up and down stairs twice a day, or before I have choked. Might I suggest she is lazy?

Overall, the interview was a catastrophe of proportions to the failed Schlieffen Plan and the resultant 16 million dead. (Go on, look it up, you know you're interested!) The above was just my impression. No doubt my Mum has further insight, as she was on translation duties for longer than I.

Of course, one has to look at the positive aspect; she left! But even that was buggered up as the driver abandoned her with us from 12.30 until 5 pm. It was four hours and 25 minutes too long.

I do not know what will happen next. Mum is trying to sort out something that will work. We all live and learn.

The following day the agency sent another applicant for us to meet. When she arrived, Mark was ill upstairs, so I let her in and told her to sit in the lounge for a moment as Mark was poorly. She didn't sit down but immediately followed me upstairs & helped out.

Mark & I knew she was the one!

Rosalia & I shared duties looking after Mark for the next few months, but it was all too much for me, and so two more carers joined us, and I was given a rest. Robin and Nick were also brilliant, but soon Rosalia had to leave, so the boys shared the work between them. I don't know how we would have coped if we hadn't had the support of these three wonderful people.

Chapter Fifteen: Extract of a letter from Mark to his uncle Robin in Canada 31/12/2013

"Hi Robin, how are you?

A good Christmas I hope and set for a jolly good New Year for 2014.

My year for 2014 does not have a high bar to jump over to be considered an improvement upon 2013. In fact, the last seven years have been very stressful with one glorious exception: Noel George Frederick Griffith born August 18th, 2010. But I have learnt rather a lot from the last few months. I can write a whole letter on that topic but, in brief, now I have a far better idea on how to really look after the stress and not just invent a façade. Many things that I have picked up from people in the very strange world I have been living in over the last year have helped me as I really shared with people during this time. Here is a bit of updating for you just in case you have not had the information yet.

On the 15th January, I will have the results given to me of the latest scan to be done on January 10th. It runs quite simply like this:-

If the three very small areas (one in neck, two in lungs that have inconclusive evidence of cancer) have gone or not grown during what will have been almost three months, then we can happily assume they are just residue from the treatment and scars that may one day go. I can carry on with my new life.

If the spot in the neck has grown then the hospital will try surgery to help me. This will mean losing my larynx completely and having to find another way of communicating. But at least I get a shot at continuing to live.

If the two small areas on my lungs have grown, then the cancer has entered the lymphatic system and given the speed & ferocity of the cancer I had/have then the doctors say they will give me a period of less than a year to continue living. Time to say goodbye to a few people.

So I start 2014 terrified if the truth were known. Normally my results from similar events end up as a mixture of outcomes, but I am not sure what the mixture of this could be. Half the problem for the specialists is that no one has ever lived as long as I have with the cancer I had/have. So they cannot make predictions as my case is unique and therefore beginning the records.

In one sense that is nice to be helpful and it seems it has proved to them that all is not lost if the patient in question is young and fit then they can up the dosage of radiation (I am not sure if the chemotherapy was increased or not). The resultant mess after the treatment is somewhat nasty, but obviously, I am still here and generally improving albeit slowly. Enough of this doom and gloom. Also, I will leave Mum to write to you on this topic as it will be therapeutic for her to talk to her brother and offload a bit of the worry closer to the results.

My Christmas was excellent as Noel stayed for a couple of nights. I have had it confirmed from his mother that he loved his time here, and I certainly did. After three years he and I became father and son and quite naturally as if we had been friends for years. In fact Father Christmas was good enough to give us both soldiers for gifts, which we both loved. Daddy could play with Noel and his military airbase for a couple of hours. He is like me in that he can make the world he is playing up in his mind very easily and from that develop whole long stories. Not destructive blow everything up immediately. Also it was lovely to see him believe that the stocking was the whole deal about Christmas. I had the pleasure of his first Christmas where he has a conscious memory and the first time he received gifts. He was not expecting and certainly not demanding. I hope this will continue for a long time.

I loved my gifts, which were mostly books or collectors models of soldiers from the First World War. I am really trying to understand the few crazy years that your father and uncles lived (and were wounded and died) through. One thing I find fascinating and almost inconceivable comes from the start and trigger of the war in August

1914. Not the assassinations or the political and nationalist background nor even the alliances that meant as one country declared war, so another had to on another country and so on and so on until almost the whole world was at war within itself. No far more basic than that and the real nuts and bolts of declaring war at that time. The massive French army is a perfect example. Once mobilization of the troops had started, it could not be halted because no one could stop the railway timetables. In fact the French had considered stopping their armies and reconsidering, but it was too late as the railway system was in operation and their troops would end up on the front lines whether they wanted it or not. Although the Germans had not considered stopping their mobilization, they too were at the mercy of the rail network at those last crucial hours before the world lost 37 million people dead and wounded. This was the crazy start to four years of murderous mayhem in which part of our family put themselves.

I can easily complete the entire letter on this one topic (the Christmas with Noel) but for you, it will end up in a repeat as Mum will really want to write about this subject to you and that is, without doubt, a grandmother's duty to keep the great uncle up to date with family events for young Noel. Suffice to say on my behalf he was very happy, and he has benefited by forming stronger bonds with his father but also grandparents, aunt, and uncle.

It is an interesting point you made about the hospital and being involved with it in some way. I have been in discussion with one of the few trachy specialist nurses and have agreed to go with her to be part of the training programme for initially the ambulance staff. It involves me being a live dummy. This is so open to all forms of hilarity that the training should become quite popular. In addition I have spent so long in so many places throughout the hospital that I know a good number of the staff. For example quite a few ambulance crew came to my home for the opening of my new shed that a charity supporting me provided.

But I am able to enjoy something, which can be seen by other participants and often spreads in a small training group, so they all learn from the course, as opposed to nodding off with boring pictures. Fortunately I am used to my trachy being changed so it can be done without it being a danger to me if mistakes are made when they practise. I now breathe through my nose and mouth as well as my trachy. All in all it looks like a win, win situation. People learn more on a live dummy, and I am back into the place.

You raised the point about visitors who are helpers. Generally the hospital does well for volunteer visitors for people in my opinion. But of course it depends upon your point of view as you enter hospital. If you embrace it as another bundle of laughs and attend with huge bright yellow slippers in the design of Homer Simpson and force the dinner ladies to read out the menu to you in a sensual style even though you have been unable to eat for a year, then you will enjoy it and spread that enjoyment. And just because you are unable to talk does not mean that the gents toilet cannot be your office with a big sign on the door just before the consultants do their very important tour at 9 am or the family visitors come in at 11 am. Also jousting matched on wheelchairs should occur at least twice a week and so on. A behind the scenes careful check on one's inmates is necessary to check what can be done and an adherence to curfew should be kept. Common courtesy to the other long timers is vital as we all have to stick together and still do now after the treatment and we are into long-term recovery or saying farewell. That approach I have mentioned also amuses and makes the place more homely for short-timers and the staff themselves. They have to deal with the more common approach of more or less nothing just sitting around feeling a bit gloomy and so making hospital a chore. These people throw up for a week and go home, which is safe but has no overall benefit for anyone. Rather like playing cards but in there we all know we have a duff hand so the only chance is to have a laugh and gamble the last chance that you get 21 and can stick.

I was told the approach I went for helped save me. Given there was nothing else left to try on me that may well have been true? It was either that or the fact that they had to get me off the ward and out of hospital before Sister murdered me!"

When Mark returned to the hospital for his next consultation, he was told the tumour on his neck had grown very slightly. The doctor suggested that if there were any travelling he had thought of doing, it would be best to do it within the next three months as his health might well deteriorate by then.

Chapter Sixteen: Battlefields Tour

Mark and I had often spoken of visiting the Battle-fields of Flanders as my father, and his three brothers had all fought in WW1. One of them had died as a result of wounds inflicted while fighting at Brettoneaux and was buried at St. Sever Cemetery in France.

I contacted Leger Holidays whose tours we had already decided covered the area we were interested in and explained the situation regarding Mark's health and asked if it would be possible for us to travel with them. They were so helpful in everything and soon we were packing our bags for our longed for holiday – All Quiet on the Western Front.

Because of the severity of Mark's condition we had his carer with us. Mark was unable to eat or drink except through a tube in his stomach but Nick, his carer, was brilliant. He had to cart a rucksack, containing all Mark's medication, everywhere and on occasions his wheelchair, although Mark tried to walk as much as possible. Our coach driver was so attentive without detracting from the pleasure of the holiday for the other passengers.

We took a day out from the tour to visit the grave of my uncle. I had arranged it through the War Graves Commission in London who had someone to meet us at the cemetery and take us to the grave. Mark was able to write in the Book of Remembrance and so record his visit.

Mark wrote a letter to each of our family to be opened after his death. There was one passage in my letter, which I would like to pass on.

'In fact, it was Thinking of dreams come true and completing my dream list, which it seems I did, you managed to complete the most important dream for me with the trip to Belgium and to walk through the trenches and to be at the Menin Gate. To get to Ypres and the Somme and stand where all the history happened some 100 years ago takes my breath away and refuels my imagination. Then to find the grave of your uncle was the icing, cherry and candles on top of the cake. Please thank all at Leger Holidays for a memorable journey'.

On returning to Norwich Mark appeared to pick up an infection and was rushed to hospital. While undergoing an MRI scan he had a massive epileptic fit and on recovery he had lost his memory. In fact he had travelled back in time some ten years and on awakening, he didn't recognise us. He thought he had been in an accident in Bulgaria and was talking about people he knew in Bulgaria (in fact he was unable to speak and so was writing this down). He was last there 10 years ago when he was working for the Foreign Office. He could remember nothing of today. This was so scary.

Karen showed him a video of Noel she had on her mobile phone – firstly he didn't remember he had a son but secondly he was intrigued with the phone – he couldn't understand how you could have a video on a phone! It took three of us several days to bring back his memory by showing him photos of family and friends.

In fact, it was a photo, taken just a few days previously on his birthday, when he recognised his cousin Glenys and from then on things seemed to be back to normal.

When Mark was safely home again, his dad suggested he might like to think about the highlights of his life and to put them in writing.

Chapter Seventeen: Highlights of My Life

Oddly enough, one of my first ever memories is Mum stepping on my model dustmen[43], breaking one and not immediately apologising. It was the floor of the kitchen in Bristol so it must be one of the earliest things that I can recall. The reason it's a highlight is that it was the first time I realised Mum was not perfect and did not apologise all the time. I was too young to know I was being a bloody nuisance!

Other very early recollections are visiting with Granddad and Grandma. Being with him in his garden, burning rubbish and garden debris. I loved the smell of that, and him showing me his greenhouse. Even better was the area beneath the greenhouse. That had a really fantastic smell and was very exciting. I played with the gnomes in the garden, the toolbox in the kitchen and the tools in the garage. Even the TV was fun because the ITV channel was completely different[44]. Granny had the 'real' Ribena drink, and her record collection was great fun. Christmas was good because the tree was different,

---

[43] Now known as Waste Technicians, more commonly called 'Bin Men' in the UK.

[44] In the 1970s, there were 3 TV channels available in the UK, two run by the BBC and the other ITV (Independent Television). ITV was regionalised on a franchise basis, with each company responsible for their own programming. Peak time slots were often identical, but there was considerable variation elsewhere in the regional schedules.

and Granny made a castle with the mashed potato. There were sausage soldiers in the towers and a moat of beans. Driving in Granddad's car was exciting too because it was shiny and smelt good. We went to Richmond Park to see the squirrels and the deer. There was a day with Grandma going to her school and a trip with Uncle Roger in his 'A' reg car[45] listening to him talking about his job at the recored company.

These all counts in my world as highlights as I remember these little things so vividly. I liked them so much that I often find myself thinking of them now.

Christmases in the lounge in Burghley Street were also highlights. The whole day was always brilliant. It started with the stocking and the same type of presents each year; the comic, the fruit, and the little toy soldiers. I loved it. Then it was off to church, where we had been the evening before at midnight, bringing in Christmas day. On the day, we could sing the one extra verse of one particular carol as well, which I always loved to do. Back home afterwards for my favourite meal of the year. Even if everyone said that the turkey was dry, I always loved it that day, come what may. The crackers with their stupid jokes, and the masses of food were all fantastic. The afternoon was spent opening all the presents in order, as slowly as possible. Of course, Dad guessed

---

[45] The Registration system for motor vehicles in the UK is based on a lettering system. The author is inferring this was a brand new car.

each of his, and Mum got a year's supply of tights all wrapped up in different parcels to keep them a secret. Karen and I always got the most ludicrous presents from the Great Aunts and Uncles, but it was all part of the special day.

While I do recall bits of my experience at playgroup, it is, of course, the enormity of my first day of real school that is a highlight. Sitting in a corridor waiting for some form of registration, I was sat with Stephen, who turned out to be the rogue of the class. Luckily, I met Jeremy, and he was my best friend for so many years. That was a close shave. But I had obviously developed the ability to differentiate between good and bad people, even at that young age. Well done Mum and Dad. We were all in Mrs. Grey's class. She smelt funny, but the sand pit was great fun. The rest of my school career at Park Road was supervised by Mrs. Peregrine, who I thought was attractive by the age of six. All girls became attractive to me, and I do not recall the age where they were not. My son has no hope!

I remember being proud of standing up in front of the class and multiplying 6 x 9 correctly. We had to have all our multiplication tables learned off by heart even by the age of six, right up to the number 12. The Christmas nativities were fun. Going to Miss Thompson's house for extra writing assignments. Mr. Spring was my first headmaster. He was in possession of a large collection of wartime memorabilia. He was history mad, and that's where I get it from. I owe him a lot for all the pleasure that has brought into my life.

The other headmaster also made quite an impression. His name was Mr. Parry. I beat up some poor little chap called Brian over a marbles game on a drain cover. We were playing for big stakes! Mr. Parry was not amused. 'I am surprised at you of all people, Mark.' Hand out and here comes the cane! Stopped me doing that again. Mind you; I had already ended up with a bloody nose from the odd fight I'd had in the park. Dad taught me to use another policy: talking and making friends (which has served me well throughout the years). It also helped to have a big best friend like Jeremy Parker, but it was from back then that I set out to be nice to the world. Well done Dad! The only time I hit anyone again was him. When I was drunk. The lowest point in my life that I can recall, but it is a 'light' in a way. A lowlight.

I also made great efforts to sit next to Mandy. Fortunately, she was smart, and they used to sit the top students together, so I had to study hard to get next to her! It was the only reason I did it. True. The school was also home to the bearded devil, Mr. Sawford. He attacked all the students. He got me to bend over and hit my bottom with a cricket bat. I went flying forward headfirst into a brass door handle. That stopped him for a while.   Just imagine that happening now!

I loved Burghley Street in general, and the Church and all the clubs. I was the minister's son, and my mother ran the massive drama club, so I was hugely proud of both of them. My sister…of course I loved her. Who else would share our hidden den in the trees where we buried Dad's dinners? Who else would share the go-cart 'Speedy' when we played in that massive garden? One highlight has to be the day I managed to stay upright on the red bike. 'Look, Dad, I'm riding the bike!' It wasn't great timing on my part as he was sat in the garden with one of his parishioners who was obviously being counselled. I spun precariously around in constant danger of crashing into walls, bushes, trees or the two of them. But I made it.

One other highlight was the first time I went to the cinema. Dad took me. The film was 'Bedknobs and Broomsticks'. I loved it. I bet I was not much more than five years old. There's a little challenge for someone; see when that film was released.[46] Something else that often comes to mind is the success I had flying a little red motorised plane in the playing field at the bottom of our road opposite the factory. I have no idea why that thought stays with me. I enjoyed flying the kitcs as well, especially the controlled ones.

---

[46] 1971. In a curious, and previously unrealised, coincidence this was also the Editor's first cinematic experience.

Another little highlight was swimming at Kettering baths. Mum always took us, and I loved it, especially the chocolate machine at the end. When we came out with our hair still damp and smelling of Chlorine, Mum would treat us to a chocolate. She also gave us fish & chips when Dad was away on trips. They were so delicious that, in hindsight, it's probably just as well he was not away for long.

I loved the next bike that I got. To me, it was a beautiful machine. My Dad showed me how to change the wheel, chain, punctures, and it had gears. We all went cycling around the countryside together. Mum had a bad knee, though, so she had a moped and I recall that Karen sat on the back. Please tell me I am mistaken in recalling she was wearing the yellow site helmet, and not a proper crash hat?

When we moved to Norwich, I still remember cycling to the caravan site to meet with Stephen. There and back. I loved that as well. Another little highlight.

The caravan holidays are all highlights in my life. Sleeping in the bunk bed with the amazing big bottom farting Karen. What a laugh. And both of us loved the sound of the rain on the roof and watching the raindrops run down the window. Having races with them. Dad getting the police channel on that big radio of ours. Of course, finding the cats. And the sun was amazing.

The summer of 1976 was a highlight all of its own. East Runton beach; building huge dam systems around the rock pools against the outgoing tide. Building massive sandcastles, which we stood on when the sea came in. Playing French cricket taught to us by the Liggins family. Searching for rabbits on the cliff tops. Going for long walks along the cliffs and to the Roman camp. The love that Karen had for such walks!!!!! Looking over the old army artillery camp on the cliffs with Mr. Storey. Long drives with Mum, navigating the map of Norfolk. Finding old air force camps there and in Northamptonshire. The late night swimming. The walks along Sheringham promenade and dodging the massive waves. The beautiful swirly ice creams. Starlings Toy Shop and my soldier collection. Playing soldiers at both caravan camps. Chips eaten from newspapers. I can still taste them now. And Pretty Corner[47] was another little highlight. I am sure all these memories cover more than just that record-breaking heatwave summer of 1976.

Holidays with my cousin Glenys were also fabulous. I think they can best be summed up by playing pirates on that boating lake. What fun we had! Mum was nigh on gasping her last by the end of it, and Karen was quite certain of yet another soaking. There was crazy golf as well, and the swing we found near the railway track.

---

[47] A beauty spot near Sheringham on the North Norfolk coast.

And why did Karen always fall into the deepest rock pools, the worst stinging nettles, and the most difficult gorse bush to rescue anyone from?

Then there were the holidays on the caravan site at Kelling Heath. It was a massive adventure. One highlight was building the fence and gate. Dad and I just went into the woods, chopped up fallen trees and dragged them back to assemble that wonderful fence. We also collected lots of stones from the beach to turn the bank into a rockery. I had a little pocketknife to 'sharpen' my stick. In those woods, I could be Robin Hood, or a Roman soldier, or whatever I wanted. Other memorable moments included swimming the mile in a little pool, and riding around with Timothy on the red two person bikes. We'd eat scampi and chips in the little bar area of the clubhouse, and I loved phoning Mum from wherever we were on the coin operated phone boxes.

As you can tell, I loved those holidays. When I was a little older, we went walking in the Lake District and The Dales. Those trips were amazing. The sense of achievement in completing those expeditions was one thing, but it was also about being with Dad. Going into a Youth Hostel and finding our own bunks, then cooking our own breakfast in the morning. It's the best fry up ever because you're ravenous, but also keen to get your boots on the ground and start walking. Dad and I climbing up some godforsaken Tor in the freezing rain, and sheltering behind a stonewall drinking black coffee from our flask. The Coast-to-Coast walk brings back some happy and funny memories too, but the times alone with Dad were my favourite. The scenery was always fantastic, no matter what the weather, but, above everything else was that glow of accomplishment.

Back home, given my father's vocation, as a family we were heavily involved with the church on London Road. One of the first things I remember about that was when Karen and I were very young; we were often asked to pick up all the little communion glasses and take them to the kitchen to be cleaned. So we drank all the remains of the Ribena[48] that was in them. I used to love that. It also led to my first paid job, of which I was very proud. I was in charge of general maintenance and door opening at weddings. I was paid 50 pence per wedding. On Saturdays sometimes there were as many as four ceremonies, which meant some rapid sweeping up of confetti, and clearing hymn books from the pews, and the like. Those wages bought me some excellent toy soldiers that even today stand proudly in my front room, and will go to my son, Noel when he's old enough. This instilled a sense of pride in doing a good job, which was very useful in the future. Thanks, Dad.

---

[48] A blackcurrant cordial originating in the UK.

I was also an active member of the local Cub Scouts. A man called Robert was Akela[49]. 'Come here, you bad boy! Akela smack botty!' Sounds questionable now, but this was in the days before perverts, and he never actually raised a hand against any of us anyway. Every year we were entered in an international competition of athletic, and various games against other Cubs from the area and some who had come over from America. Robert assumed that our team would not win because none of his teams ever did, but he just told us to go ahead and do our best. Well, we won, and his face was even happier than ours. He took us all out for a meal in a restaurant somewhere as a treat. I have never seen a happier man. That was a real highlight for me.

There were several youth clubs connected to the church. I enjoyed running around the table tennis table and playing the 'killer' at snooker. But what I loved was staying over at Nassington. It's a small village west of Peterborough, and kids went there for activities like canoeing. Messing around on the water was great, but what I was even better was the night game. We were scattered throughout the countryside and had to get back to the base without being caught. I often remember that and smile to myself. Again, something that could not happen today.

---

[49] Cubmaster or Den Leader; adult supervisor of the pack.

Mum also ran the drama club. Every production had its highlights of love and little disasters. It was during one of these productions that I asked a girl out for the first time, and she said yes. I was heartbroken to receive a letter from her father, telling me that she was too young. Our first production was Pinocchio, and I played the lead. Listening to the applause and seeing my Mum's face smiling at us, was a joy I shall always treasure. Especially considering she had wanted to kill us for being so hopeless in rehearsals. From that moment on, I had no fear of speaking in public and the benefits from that confidence have been untold. In fact, it's made me who I am. For that, I am very grateful to my Mum. I have been able to help so many people by just standing and being unafraid to speak out. By being able to take positive action, whether in teaching or in diplomacy.

The other role that springs to mind was playing John in Peter Pan. The flying was brilliant, of course, but I also loved the cast. Timothy played my brother; Robert was the Pirate, Captain Hook, and Mandy was Peter Pan. It was a great combination, and everyone else was fantastic too. Of all the shows we did, I think that was my favourite overall. Playing a soldier with Jeremy in Robin Hood was great fun as well.

As a side product of all this, my parents took me to shows in London, including Peter Pan. I loved seeing shows. Other highlights were 'The Mousetrap' and the trip we made for my parent's anniversary. On that occasion, the added humour of the lunch box gay snack bar was a particular delight. I have many happy memories of the drama group, and I was so very proud that it was my Mum who was in charge, and that I was the 'boss's son'.

After we had moved to Norwich, there are fewer highlights, even though I enjoyed the clubs that I joined. Maybe that is an age thing. But there were some happy moments during those five years. I recall celebrating Mum's birthday at a Greek restaurant in East Runton. The surprise was fantastic as lots of family and relatives were there. Mum's face was a picture. Of course, it was during this time that I had my first real girlfriend and my first broken heart. As I look back now, I realise why some of my wives were idiots. It seems I have always based my romantic decisions on an initial choice of love or lust!

As far as school went, the holidays with the choir to Vienna were worthy of note. I loved the city, and the coffees were fantastic. The trips to Sonnenburg and the ridiculous fun we had there were wonderful too, but little else stands out from that time. It seems a shame almost. But I loved my job at Greens in Debenhams outside of school hours, perhaps because I'd found it myself and worked there so long.

My holiday trip on the trains around Europe was also very special. I met a wonderful range of people and slept in some very odd places. At one point, I arrived in a quiet town in Spain at the end of the line in the Basque region. No one spoke English, but I got a full meal of various foods that the occupants of a bar wanted me to try. I was just sitting in the loo getting rid of some of it when the place went crazy. I assumed a bomb had gone off, or a revolution had started. No, it was a three-day carnival, which it seemed to me had been organised while I was having a quiet poo! I ended up spending my time with a Spanish bullfighting team who did not have a bull and only knew one English word: 'friend'. It was a great couple of days. I slept in someone's house and got fully organised just using the word 'friend'. I made out with a beautiful Norwegian girl on top of a large hill in that wonderful countryside. Given that I had originally spotted her in France on a beach, that was pretty amazing.

There were other highlights on that trip. Meeting up with Dad in Norway, and staying up all night in the sunlight drinking his Christmas beer. Sleeping on the steps of Venice railway station for a couple of days and living off the pizza from the trolley outside the main gate. That city was lovely, and a friend and I enjoyed sending Americans the wrong way around the tiny map of the canal system that the various hotels supplied. Very happy moments.

College does not hold any standout moments other than watching the Royal Tattoo[50] from the lighting stalls with an RAF mechanic. He took me up there to sit and watch it all. We had a great laugh, and ate all the free hot dogs that I was supposed to be selling! That might explain why I was wheeling around beef at my next assignment: Crufts. It was enjoyable being a 'real' student, though, with all the stupid parties and pranks. Those jokes will not be forgotten. The house I stayed in was only really memorable for the level of filth that we created. Even the mice left in disgust! Graduation was not a highlight either. I guess some of my female conquests of the time were wonderful, but looking back now, it was just the start of a history of great affairs and disastrous marriages. None of my marriages are highlights.

The following year after college I went to live with Granny. Uncle Martin was also in residence. He created what became known as the six-month curry. It was a sight to behold, and a wonder to taste. It cooked over the lowest gas for week after week after week. There was also our trained squirrel. He became a pet, and would come into the kitchen to visit. Until that fateful day when he escaped into the hallway and ran into Granny. She went mental. I received the historical dressing down of all time. So did Martin. I suspect that the squirrel's escape was the beginning of the end of our stay.

---

[50] A military performance of music or display by the armed forces.

My first real job as a Quantity Surveyor is definitely not something I regard as a high point, and the Channel Tunnel job was just another job, and really rather boring. That phrase rather sums up that little spell of my life, but it was followed by working at the prison and shouting down the big, black leader of the class. I humiliated him in front of his peers, and never had a problem working there for the next two years. Even when classes changed, the respect remained. The big hug I got from a mother in the middle of a shop in Balham for helping her boy steer his life away from crime into a regular job in the building trade. Sadly, it may have been my only success in the time I was there, but helping even one person was something.

I really enjoyed working with the Foreign Office and saw so many famous people that it ceased to be anything close to unusual, just part of a routine. I guess the impromptu meeting with President Clinton was a highlight. The five minutes we chatted while staring at the erect nipples of a young female colleague in a white top was very funny. The beautiful houses I got to work in like Chequers were pretty special. When I got the full-time job with the Foreign Office and was told that over 2,000 people had applied for each position was not too shabby either. Better than my graduation.

My first job overseas was a highlight. Travelling to Bulgaria, the wonderful flat, the great new friends I made. Nothing beats that. I even managed to ignore the idiot wife who immediately started moaning about everything. She ended up with a job she liked outside of my life, so that was that, save for the odd meeting. Of course, the problems resurfaced when I was posted elsewhere.

Out of all the fun and hard work in Bulgaria, it is difficult to pick out high points, but I'll try. I did a lot of consular duty with a woman named Hilary. We both hated football but had to look after a Chelsea vs. Sofia match. We handed out free tickets to all our drivers and our Management Officer Gary, making them temporary consular officers. The looks on their faces were priceless. Better still was the fact that Hilary and I had to make an HQ away from the game, but remain in radio contact with all of these guys in case of trouble. So we set up in the local pub with the TV on in the background!

Trying to put together Karl's indoor gym assisted by two bottles of rare port and a huge lump of rarer cheese from his diplomatic bags was so funny. Our abject failure and consumption of all his precious supplies was hilarious, if not to him. Karl also taught me to ski. I did manage to get some of the basics down thank heavens, but he failed to understand why I found falling over all the time so funny. My fellow student was a guy called Aurea. He just couldn't get it at all. Karl was furious. How could someone fail to understand a fully trained commando ski instructor? Aurea was the first. It was so funny to watch.

Working with Gary was a privilege, and the trip to Thailand for his wedding was fantastic. The north of the country is beautiful, and the wedding was truly unique. We all took a special part in the ceremony, and monks officiated. Plus the curries there were seriously hot. The birth of his first child is also a special memory.

I also met the woman of my dreams, so Billyanna has to have a quick mention as it's not often the most beautiful woman on earth kisses you.

I had many great holidays, and I have to admit my first wife did us proud there. Although, I had to pay for everything, of course! There were a number of great business trips, too; Istanbul, the historical sights in Israel, the rainforest in New Zealand, the Grand Canyon in America. There were so many beautiful places in Greece as well. Managing to get Mum up to the top of the Acropolis remains a victory for the both of us.

Getting to the rain-sodden island of Kefalonia and seeing Dad's noncommittal face after all the travel I had done was funny in its own right. That holiday was classic, what with the flooded restaurants and Karen's fighting friends. But it did lighten up when Mum and I left the others and climbed over the hill into the town. The pair of us were always the adventurous types. That was a lovely day.

The civil war started when I was in Khartoum, and I had to arrange the evacuation of the Embassy. I got shot at, but I managed to get everyone out, including all the children of the locally engaged staff. I was proud of myself for that. The thanks I got was nil but who really cares? I did my job and more, literally under fire. Keeping the family tradition going.

In Albania, I personally paid for the first ever staff party at the Embassy for the locally engaged staff. They were so happy. I also helped one of my staff with her dissertation for her Masters on the European Union. She passed and her pleasure was infectious. Despite all that, I was a huge fraud in the eyes of my employer. So, while it's a sad highlight, it was one nevertheless when the jury delivered their unanimous 'not guilty' to the charges that remained in that crazy court case.

My job at County Hall in Norwich brought no highlights, apart from all the friends that I made. The flat I lived in when I moved back to Norfolk and the house that I've bought are both highlights to me. I loved the flat and love this home.

As you may have worked out by now, I've been taking these in historical order, so now we come to my son Noel. I remember holding him for the first time after his birth in the hospital. My father was standing right next to me at the time; three generations of the men in the Griffith family. I am sure someone took a photograph, which I would love to see again and perhaps frame.

When Noel was still quite young, but walking, I managed to get him alone and took him to the park near the flat. I 'left' my phone at home under the bedcovers, so no one was certain where we had escaped to. Especially as we went to the rear of the park where the massive slide is. I was so proud of my son as he ran up this slide and slid down. He kept me running up and down the slide or kicking our football up it, and running after it, for the best part of an hour. The other fathers were impressed; I was knackered.

The day with him at Lowestoft beach with Mum and Dad is very special to me. Just the four of us. I have the photograph in my front room of just me and him by the water's edge. I really enjoyed that day and was so proud of my son and the way he joined in with others so easily. Just like his father. He laughed as he threw himself into the sea and got so absorbed in his games. Again just like his father.

Then there was Noel's first Christmas here. Looking at his face when he unwrapped each toy, especially the fort. But his assumption that not everything was his was a wonderful thing to see. There is no selfishness in him at all. Seeing him playing at East Runton beach like I used to do was a wonderful sight. Likewise, the day at the Dinosaur Park[51] was great fun in its own right, but seeing how strong and brave the young lad was with the rope ladders and the slides made me proud of him, as well.

Happy highlights include the day when I came out of the hospice to see Noel at home, and the back garden had been done up for me. I think another highlight will be when the whole garden is complete, front and back, and even the patio. The battlefields holiday in Belguim that Mum arranged for me was another standout. I can think of that every day, and it still makes me smile. I am so happy that I managed that with Mum and my carer, Nick. Being at the Menin Gate, walking through trenches at Ypres, finding my great uncles' grave and standing with Nick at Hawthorn Ridge just remembering the massive explosion and the start of the Somme offensive. We were standing where history was made. After the trip, Mum and I began buying model soldiers and creating a Great War scene.

---

[51] The Dinosaur Adventure Park in Lenwade, Norfolk.

To bring things right up to date, I spent last Saturday afternoon with Dad playing with the train set for Noel and then in the evening I played 'Diplomacy'[52] with Mum. Some highlights are just so simple to achieve. I've also loved being with my sister, listening to her stories of idiots at work. I hope that talking about it helps to relieve her frustration.

I am not so sycophantic as to say that each day of my life now is a highlight because that is just not true. But I do know I still have highlights to come, so this list will always remain a work in progress.

[52] A popular American board game.

Chapter Eighteen: Ten examples of Visa Applications I handled when working overseas for various British Embassies

In 2006, the average refusal rate for worldwide entry to the United Kingdom was just 19% of all applications. My refusal rate was 84%. I believe that I had the highest refusal rate in the world at that point. So, if you came into my office with your application and sat on the other side of the bulletproof glass, your chances of success were not great. Having said that, I did take most difficult cases, simply because someone had to. If the applicant did not speak English, I had a translator immediately render their pearls of wisdom in my native tongue. I was always very pleasant to my customers. Some of them were not ready for this, and so fell into my trap. They actually told the truth.

Here are ten instances of classic applications, in no particular order:

1. Football Mania

This idiot had tried and failed, to get into the United Kingdom on several occasions. He was a Bulgarian with no money, and no skills to offer a prospective new homeland. The other slight problem was that I knew that his brother was working illegally in Britain already. So, the idea of giving him a visitor's visa was out of the question.

His application, this time, was based on his love of football, particularly Manchester United. He had to go to a match in the U.K. to see his heroes play. He was so much of a fan that he had legally changed his name to Manchester United. Yes, I had to interview Manchester United, who wanted to visit Great Britain to see Manchester United.

This lunatic had also managed to get the Sun newspaper to back him, and try to pressure me into allowing it out of sympathy. What do you think happened to Manchester United? Correct. He picked up another refusal to add to his collection, and he got to remain in Bulgaria until it became part of the European Union. Manchester United is no doubt in the U.K. by now. Possibly running some dubious business. Possibly in Manchester.

2. The Curse

Some people really got annoyed with me when I refused them. There was an old and wrinkly-faced gipsy woman from a village far up in the mountains of Bulgaria. She had travelled many days to get to me. Probably on a knackered old donkey. She had brought her entire family with her. It was obvious that they assumed I would simply issue her the visa, and they would head down the road, selling heather as they went, until they stumbled upon the airport with the big silver bird that would whisk her off to her new life in the promised land. She was going to live with her daughter and look after the grandchildren. A fine plan. Unfortunately, it would be allowing her daughter to work. And that would be illegal because the daughter was in the country illegally in the first place. Then the whole family could benefit from the free health care and services paid for by the taxes of everyone who actually had a right to live there. The list of crimes was starting to build, but it all seemed perfectly fine to my suddenly not so friendly gipsy.

She was refused the Entry Clearance and went berserk. She started frothing at the mouth, spat at the glass, and hurled all forms of abuse at me. Once she had left and we had dug the chair back out of the wall (exaggeration!), my interpreter informed me that I had been given a powerful gipsy curse. Ha! I said. Now, I have to wonder. It's two violent marriages later with me as the victim, and a massive loss of money on both occasions. My last wife was arrested and convicted because she attacked me. She was even too mad for Norwich. And there's the terminal cancer, of course. So, as I say, I do have to wonder. If I'd turned a blind eye just that once…

3. Fraudulent Behaviour

Of course, you have all heard of how diplomats can be offered bribes. On occasion, this can involve large sums of money. Well, this happened to your own friendly little diplomat. Shocking but true revelations are about to follow!

There I was in Albania faced with another wizened old person hoping for a visa to get into the UK to visit his son. And lo! The Archangel came down, and there was much light and happiness. Because the son was in the UK legally, and with a very decent job. This old man was his real father, and he had not lied on his application form. This was a very difficult thing for an Albanian to do. The father had no reason to remain in the UK afterwards so, for once, I was going to have an easy time with all the paperwork and give him the clearance he needed.

Then the inherent lunacy of the country popped its head up over the parapet. A very smelly piece of paper was pushed under the window of the glass barrier. It smelt of tobacco that had been made from the leaves of a potato plant and then wrapped around a dead donkey's lower regions that should never be named. Or, alternatively, it had been used several times in a lavatorial emergency in a bad Albanian toilet. At first, I assumed it to be a weapon of chemical warfare and began the Embassy evacuation alert, but then I recognised it as currency. My translator explained that I was being offered it so that I would look kindly on his application. Look kindly on it! It was more likely I would throw up on it. He was hoping that I would give him the Entrance Clearance and risk my entire career for the equivalent of five and a half pence.[53]

It was a significant amount of money to that old man. It was sad. He broke the law just seconds before being given exactly what he wanted. I asked the translator to explain that his action was a serious violation of our law, wrapped up the note with a piece of paper from my pocket, and stuffed it back under the window. He left with £11.

4. The Honeytrap

We all recall moments in the James Bond films where the sexy woman comes into his room wearing nothing but a fur coat, which she drops at the sight of him to get at his secrets. We were even trained to expect this sort of behaviour, especially in Eastern Europe where I worked for ten years. Discounting my last marriage, this is the story of the one time in a decade that it actually happened to me.

---

[53] Approximately 8 Cents in US currency.

I was sat on my own in an empty restaurant just after work waiting for some Bulgarian friends who didn't turn up (please insert a swear word of your own choice regarding these ex-friends). I would have been in my mid to late 30's then, and I guess the woman in question would have been about ten years older than that. Now, the poor dear had a nice enough figure and was not bad looking but not in the get-up she was wearing. There were thigh-high black squeaky plastic boots, black stockings, a black plastic mini skirt, black stiletto shoes, a white blouse and a red bra. I assumed that this rig came with scaffolding to help her get into it and that there were stabilisers tucked in there somewhere. It was all topped off with a fur coat, probably weasel. This fur had a head that the West End of London would have been proud of, assuming it was Christmas pantomime time!

I do not profess in any way to know the details of the mystery that is a woman's face make-up, but this was obviously DIY time. Panda eyes, eyelashes that attacked me from over two feet away and so much red on her cheeks and lips that I assumed she was drunk even before she began purchasing the gallons of wine in a feeble attempt to try and get me drunk. That was not a very sensible strategy. I was already being paid by the British Government to drink for our country. Or something like that.

The woman launched into the usual junk, asking whether she could join me. She spoke very good English. Do not ask how I knew it wasn't a whore, just take that as a fact. Considering the speed with which she sat and the first vat of wine had arrived, my answer regarding her request would have been irrelevant. There was about six seconds of general chitchat until she came straight to the point. If I gave her daughter a student visa, I would get rumpty pumpty with her. And this was a mere taster of further delights to come. Assuming her daughter would have been about 18, I made a rough guess as to what those would be, and where my preference would lie in a different world.

But, back to reality. I could have taken advantage. It would hardly have been a great fall into a pit of forbidden pleasure, more like a stumble on a kerb stone really. But I was no James Bond. I did the only thing a sensible man could do in a situation like that. I told her to shut up. She burst into tears, and I realised that I wasn't a sensible man, after all. Her face fell apart and released quite a pleasant human being. Once the ladies toilet had been used as her changing room again, we had a chat. I explained the obvious. Her daughter needed to make an application!

She told me that her husband was in the UK, working legally. She showed me a photograph of a man who had fists the size of my head. Another good reason for not being stupid. I managed to extricate myself from the conversation tactfully. It was not my job to listen to her confessions in a dodgy restaurant. It was up to her daughter to attend an interview at the Embassy, and I'd take it from there. Well, the daughter came in, and she did not lie on her application. There was a lot of checking, and weighing the balance of probabilities. Was it a genuine case, or not? In the end, I issued the clearance.

I received Christmas cards from the family for years afterwards, and the daughter graduated in English and another qualification. She worked both in the United Kingdom and in Bulgaria. I doubt if her mother ever mentioned her near exploit to anyone.

5. To P Or Not To P

We could be very intimidating to some poor applicants. I remember one woman who came in was so terrified that she just sat down on the stool and wet herself before she'd even uttered one word. She did not move throughout the whole interview and said virtually nothing. The pungent smell of the urine all over her skirt and the stool filled the air like a rare Albanian perfume. To be honest, I can't remember if she was refused or not. I think she was part of a tour group, so the answer was most likely a refusal. She left through the crowd. It was probably one of the worst days of her life.

6. The Crying Game

Then there was the woman who started crying about two minutes into the interview. If I remember correctly, she was applying for clearance for a family visit. Now, I am aware that some women turn on the waterworks because they believe that men will just surrender, and give them what they want. I hate people who cry for no real reason and instructed the female translator to tell her that she was potentially damaging her chances by such behaviour. She said it was nerves, and she could not stop. In the end, both myself and the translator actually believed her. So we carried on as the wailing getting worse. It got so bad in the end that the Consul himself came in and asked me what the hell did I think I was doing? God knows what the public must have thought. The noise was loud enough to be heard in the waiting room outside.

I got what information I could and the translator and I left the room, me to do some checking, her to remain listening at the door. The crying woman did not stop when she was left alone in the room. To cut a long story short, on balance, I felt that she was actually a genuine applicant. So back in we went. She was still sniffling and weeping. I tell her the good news. You guessed it. She started crying with joy. I smiled and left to try and explain to my boss why I was mistreating customers.

7. Ant Attack

Do you get really annoyed at work when technology fails? When computers freeze and crash and so on? Well, anyone who thinks life as a Diplomat working in overseas Embassies is a glamorous alternative is mad. Sure, it can be fun; take my sister's episode with hot coffee and the crotch of a British Army officer, for instance. But our workday issues can be far more basic and immediate than a malfunctioning disk drive.

Early on in my career, I was in the middle of conducting an interview with an applicant when suddenly my desk erupted with a swarm of red ants. Rather than shouting 'run for your life' I thought protocol required me to maintain the British stiff upper lip and carry on, no matter what. The translator looked to me for instructions, but I gave none, so the three of us had to sit through the rest of the interview trying to ignore the fact that we were getting covered slowly in these bloody ants.

In the end, the applicant was left to walk out dripping ants off his body, and we just ran into our main office to find ant killer and clean up. That is the closest I have ever got to appearing in a horror film.

8. A Dead Disastrous Day

I also did consular work, which means looking after the Brits abroad. There was one man who drank himself to death on the other side of Bulgaria some time before I'd arrived. He had no money, no passport, and was only known by a nickname. We'll call him Bob. When he died, there were only very limited details of where he'd lived in the UK. The Foreign Office and. British police did the usual family search but had no luck. So Bob was buried in a pauper's grave on the Black Sea. It had to be nameless because no one knew his real name. He had just arrived in Bulgaria and then spent the few years he had left getting blind drunk.

We had an Honorary Consul out there on the Black Sea coast, who we visited from time to time. We also sent him staff, especially in the summer. He needed help with the idiots on holiday who got drunk, and then get robbed. The ones who lose passports, the ones who claim rape but then realise it was just a big argument with their boyfriend, or that sleeping with the ugly waiter had seemed like a good idea at the time. Some even managed to smash something up, themselves on occasion and ended up in either hospital or prison. It wasn't nice over there. I never go on holiday abroad. It is too scary! Anyway, no one had claimed this dead Brit when I took the job over. I was told the little of his history that we knew, and his nickname and that was it.

One evening I was getting into a taxi after an exhausting trip to my local pub, and my emergency Embassy phone went. I sobered up quickly and answered. 'This is the emergency line of the British Embassy in Bulgaria. Please, can you give me the nature of your emergency?' I was waiting for the usual stuff. My husband is in jail, I have been robbed, or I am drunk and standing naked in the centre of Sofia, what do I do? But no, it was the sister of our long dead nameless Brit. 'I wonder if you know the address of my brother? He was last heard of living near the Black Sea. He is a bit of a loner so you may have a problem.' She gave me his nickname, so I knew his identity immediately. I could have said; 'Actually, it's not a problem. He's six feet under a pile of earth right now.' However, I just took all the details. The police would visit her and break the news face to face, just in case she was alone and collapsed when she heard. I got back out of the cab and returned to the pub! In my defence, wife number two was horrible, so it was a much better option than returning home.

A couple of weeks went by and then the dreaded call came. Bob's family want to visit his grave to pay their respects. Of course, the Ambassador heard about it somehow and decided to make a show of it to display how good we were at public relations. So we dragged our local vicar out of the lap-dancing club and dry-cleaned both him and his clerical robes. Someone found his Bible and told him what to read. The Embassy management officer arranged for the family of six to be picked up from the airport and taken to the hotel in Sofia, which had been arranged for them. They would travel down the coast the following day at our expense, and begin their holiday. It would start with a ceremony led by our vicar at Bob's graveside.

I went across the country to the coast to see the Honorary Consul and to visit the grave in advance. As this had turned into a public relations exercise, I wanted to be sure that Bob's final resting place was clean and tidy. What a jolly surprise I got when I arrived. "Who the hell is Bob?" Oh dear. I think I sacked the Honorary Consul ten times in my reply to his question, as well as all of his staff, his family and the family of his staff. But it did not help. All anyone could remember was that there had been this drunken Brit, who had died sometime before, and was buried in a pauper's grave somewhere. Great. I knew that already. How about where? I finally got one of the locals to stop crying by telling them that I was actually a nice guy, and no one would lose their jobs if they all shut up and did exactly what I told them. She phoned the local council on my behalf. We found out, to my delight, that there was just one cemetery in the area Bob had lived that took paupers. So we legged it down there to find the grave.

Of course, it was a massive cemetery. There was much wandering about in the midday sun looking for the pauper's area and much of cursing of Englishmen who had forgotten to ask the lcoal council exactly where it was. But we found it eventually. A polite translation of my reaction when I was faced with it was 'Bloody hell'. Half the population of the Black Sea coast must have been broke, and gone there to die. There was row upon row of broken sticks in the ground, standing over little mounds of earth. Everything was covered in a jungle of weeds and nettles. I checked each little marker for a name; any name, but preferrably Bob. Nothing. They were all nameless. Bob was not in sight.

The local staff all buggered off for ice cream, which was fair enough as I had shouted at them earlier. I continued my search for Bob. What did the keeper of the cemetery know about it? Nothing. His staff? Nothing. The gravediggers? Nothing. I stared up toward heaven and wondered if Bob was known only unto God, like the Unknown Soldier. I was left with one choice. I randomly picked a grave, swore everyone to abolute silence forever, and had it cleaned up. All the neighbours got a quick shave and a tidy up as well. Bob's grave was magnificent by the time we had finished. The Commonwealth War Graves Commission would have been proud of our work. The broken marker was replaced with a more substantial post and a plaque. A quick phone call to his innocent family gave us his date of birth, and a guess at the date of death allowed for an appropriate inscription.

The entourage arrived the next day. The family wore all their best clothes, and the vicar was respendent in all his finery. Also present were the Honorary Consul, his deputy, and the Consul and Vice Consul of the British Embassy; that was my boss and me. I made the introductions and led the party slowly through the cemetery and up to the beautiful grave. The vicar said his meaningful words of condolence. Heaven only knew whose remains he was speaking over, but whoever it was got a wonderful if slightly delayed, send off to eternity. Rest in Peace, Bob!

9. World's Worst Wife

Let's go over the mountains now to the land of goat herders and general idiots. Trust me; it's a fair description of Albanians. I should know; I married one: Disaster Wife Number 3.

Working on visa applications can be a difficult decision-making process, particualrly if it concerns someone who wants to go and live in the UK forever as part of a married couple. There are a lot of emotions involved, especially if the applcants are young. The evidence required is complex, but I think the decision really comes down to one thing: is the marriage a sham or not? I had to weigh up the balalce of probabilities to reach an answer on each application.

Some marriages in Albania are a sham, almost 99% in fact. There are arranged marriages, even between Albanians, and there are many where the man marries a 16-year-old virgin and her role is merely to bear children and look after the house. This leaves him free to have all the mistresses he can afford. This is a fact. I knew many people with marriages just like that. So, when an Albanian marries an English girl, it's usually a ruse to allow him into the UK to work. If he remains married for two years, he can legally stay in the UK for the rest of his life. It doesn't matter if they subsequently divorce. So, these situations were tricky, and it was important to get the decision right. Any refusal I made had to be watertight as most refusals were appealled, and the appeal process was not robust; it favoured those making the appeal. The specific case I am going to talk about started just the same as hundreds of others; with the interview. It ended in chaos.

The Albanian man arrived in my office for our meeting, and a handsome young fellow he was. He spoke good English. I checked and found that this was because he had lived in the UK before. Illegally. But he was not thrown out of the country; he returned to Albania voluntarily. That meant he was able to reapply to go back now that he had married a UK cirtizen. I will not bore you with the Immigration Rules.

At this point, there was a knock on my door. Security wanted a word with me. The wife was outside, demanding to be involved in the interview, and her mother was there as well. This is not allowed. As I did not need my translator, I sent her out with the guard to explain and to calm things down. I returned to the interview room and started to examine the photographs that were provided with the application. Normally, they tell the whole story. I went cold and then hot and then felt sick. I have seen ugly creatures in my life, but this female came from a different planet. God, she was ugly. The husband was a builder, but she was three times his size and incredibly fat. I swear that the warts on her face had warts of their own. Where she managed to find clothes to wear, I do not know. Camping shops, I presume. Her hair was matted down and dyed two tones of off-colour blonde.

In all, there were seven photographs of their happy day. She had a cigarette permanently in her jowls where the rest of mankind would have a mouth. The body was just one lump. Nothing was obvious within it. A blessing maybe. Her rear end put many a bulldozer to shame. This load was supported by two huge tree stumps that only parted at the knees to admit a crack of daylight. I looked up at the applicant, and he just smiled back and said: 'But I love her'.

Of course, I have seen many mismatched couples in my life, and you have to be careful. You can't just write people off based on physical appearance alone, but the rest of the application was a joke. They had just seven pictures of an alleged two-year relationship. All had been taken on the same day at the same place, and it was just down the road from the Embassy. He could barely remember any details about her beyond her name, and that she did not work and lived with her mother in a Council house in North London. Answers on where they had met lacked any kind of consistency. The bank account details showed no income from anything other than benefits. So the British taxpayers would be supporting them, which was illegal under the immigration rules. It was an easy refusal.

I was about to thank him and ask him to wait outside while I considered his application when the door was removed from its hinges and hurled into my office. Suddenly, I was face to face with the snarling beast from the pits of hell. I now know what it must have been like to have run into the Blitzkrieg in 1940 in France. Stormtroopers charging at you with whole SS Panzer divisions following and Stuka dive bombers screaming in the sky above. But, unlike the French, I could not run away and surrender. I had to face it. I had nowhere to go, and I was all alone. I tried to concentrate on the one little pleasure I could get out of the situation: the verbal battering I could give our security team afterwards for allowing her in. Little did I know that they were scattered around the waiting room like rag dolls.

Her swearing went on for over five minutes and at such a volume that I thought the glass barrier between us would shatter. She was pushed right up against it, lest I should miss one of the F words or the other variations that seemed to involve the whole alphabet. The Consul opened the other door to my office. The Consul shut the other door to my office. He stayed on the other side of it. The only time I ever heard comparable language and a tirade that lasted longer was courtesy of Wife Number 3.

Eventually, she took a breath, and I was able to say. 'A pleasure to meet you, Mrs. Rhinocerous. Please take a seat. I believe it is under the door that fell off as you came in. I am so sorry about that'. Or words to that effect, anyway. I was as polite as I could be, having quickly decided that the best thing to do would be to give her an interview as genuine as her marriage. Better than risking further damage to staff or property. So I asked some feeble questions. Where had they met? A new answer. When had they met? An answer that wasn't even the same as the one provided on their application. In fact, the only information she gave that was consistent with the form was that she was unemployed, and lived with her unemployed mother in a Council house. Not one other member of the family had turned up for the 'wedding.'

Now, you may be wondering how these two creatures could afford a trip to Albania in the first place. Well, in my experience, it is amazing how much money some unemployed people actually have. How many foreign holidays can an unemployed ex-wife afford, for example? Well, I count five, if she goes to France twice in the school holidays. But I digress…

The case wasn't unfamiliar to me. I'd seen the exact set of circumstances before. A foreign national working illegally in Great Britain knows he is about to be deported by the Home Office. That means that any further application he makes to enter the country is highly likely to be automatically refused. Therefore, he needs to take drastic action; he needs to get married. So he finds a desperate British woman who has little chance of receiving a matrimonial proposal and tricks her into believing that he loves her. Or, in some cases offers her a lot of money. Then it's a quick trip for the two of them back to his home country; first to get married then to the British Embassy.

I warned all the security staff that I was going to refuse the application. It meant his only way back into the UK was in the back of a lorry. For her, it meant heartbreak because she thought it was real. The truth was that the partnership would have lasted as long as it took me to say 'I do' to the application and stamp the paperwork. But, of course, she did not know that. When I told him he was refused, he just left quietly. He'd probably guessed. Her reaction was quite different. She went completely mental and stayed in the office until closing time shouting at the top of her lungs. I left when it became obvious that it was pointless trying to explain why he had been refused. Eventually, a very brave security guard entered the rubble that had been my office and told her that everyone had gone home, and if she stayed any longer, she would have to be locked in. He ran, and lived to tell the tale. However, she did understand, and lumbered out of the office, through the public side of the consulate and left. Or so I thought!

Our office shut to the public at 4 pm, with the staff usually leaving an hour later. A few of the Brits, including myself, would often carry on until around 6 pm, and then have a couple of wines or so with colleagues in a bar on the Embassy road. We'd meet up with the French, so we could insult them, the Dutch so we could try to outdrink them, or the Italians so we could laugh at them. And so on. That particular evening I was going to meet a friend from the British army, and a friend from the British police, both of whom were working with us. It was the summer time and sunny and warm; a perfect evening to sit outside, have a chat over a drink and, in my case, avoid Wife Number 2.

I walked out of the Embassy and heard an awful shriek. 'There he is, the f***ing bastard.' I turned, and saw the distraught wife, a sad little husband trying to escape her clutches, and what can only be described as a monster that was even bigger than the daughter. It was her mother. Now, I have had bad mother-in-laws, but she beat everything. Fortunately, speed was not on their side, but they were right outside the Embassy, so my only option was a tactical retreat behind the gates. I faced another torrent of abuse. One of them had come up with the phrase 'Our human right to be married' and was trying to beat it to death. I agreed with the sentiment but thought that they had to be human to have that right, and I'd seen little evidence of that.

The Consul came out, followed by the Deputy Ambassador with security in tow. They tried to calm the women down, but the shoutng went on for ages. Eventually, there was a quiet spell, and I managed to explain to the mother that they did have the right to appeal the decision. They could write in to explain their grievance, re-apply, and another officer would interview the husband. That was an error. They jumped at the chance, despite the £800 cost. So poor were these unemployed people! Then the Consul mentioned that the length of the queue was six months. To say they were not happy was the understatement of many decades. I thought we were in for an episode of the 'Incredible Hulk', but then they were ugly and massive already. Just not green.

I could sense that the Consul was going to cave in and overturn my decision just to stop all the grief. So I had a quiet word with the Deputy Ambassador. She was a fan of my work, and I thought highly of her. I explained the history of the husband with regards to his residence in the UK. The Immigration Officers at Gatwick would have a field day with us if they spotted him trying to get back into the country. Anyone who signed the papers would be in a lot of trouble. She understood. And I bribed her with a bottle of wine, provided we made it out alive, of course. She took them on verbally for a few minutes, but we were still trapped behind the gate with two real live gargoyles yelling obscenties at us.

Now, I am not exaggerating the next bit. My friends could see there was a problem from where they were sitting in the restaurant. This road had seven embassies on it, plus some accommodation for visiting diplomats. It was a possible terrorist target, so there were barriers and armed guards at either end. The British Army friend went one way, and the policeman the other. They told each troop that we were under attack. So six guards came running up armed with a machine gun, a semi-automatic rifle and four handguns.

None of the soldiers spoke English. They did not need to. With this arsenal facing them, the weeping bride, her infuriated mother, and the bedraggled husband beat a swift retreat. My debt went up to six bottles of beer for the guards, and a couple of pints each for my friends in the police and army.

To complete the story, some time later a few scraps of paper appeared on my desk. It was their appeal. Reading it, I realised that the husband had done a runner anyway. They weren't able to contact him, and he'd probably given them a false address anyway. I wrote my reply and sent the bundle off to the appeal appellate. They were refused some six months later. Gentlemen, I warn you: Beware of North London!

10. My 'Basil Fawlty' Interview

One last gem; this one from Bulgaria.

There are a few things that I hate. Women crying for no real good reason and my last two ex-wives for instance. But perhaps my greatest hatred is reserved for people using the phrase 'It is My Right'. No, it is not. You do not have a right without a duty; be that of care or to your country, or whatever. You cannot, as far as I am concerned, just have a right without earning it in some way. You may be surprised to know that I don't think unemployed people have a right to benefits without having first paid taxes, and/or be actively and seriously looking for work. Not buggering about on holidays where the taxpayers foot the bill.

I acknowledge that I'm not working at the moment, but I have spent the last 30 years in gainful employment. Firstly, as a student on weekends, holidays or during University years and then permanently as a Quantity Surveyor, a teacher, a diplomat, and finally as even I don't know what at County Hall in Norwich. I have paid a good deal of income tax and National Insurance. I will now get off my soapbox, but there was a reason for that little rant. It shows you how strongly I feel about such matters.

One afternoon I was in my little office with my interpreter. It had been a normal day spent refusing people the chance to change their lives at the expense of the UK taxpayer. Then a woman arrived who wanted to join her husband and family in the UK. The stumbling block was that he had originally entered and worked in the country illegally. His status had now been straightened out to some extent, but it wasn't straightforward, and the Immigration Rules were complicated. I won't bore you with all the details.

The bottom line was that I needed to ask her the right questions and get satisfactory answers. Unfortunately, this lady had come in with the attitude that the interview was procedure, and just a boring little piece of bureaucracy that was not just in the way of her move to the UK, it was in the way of her day. She just kept interrupting, and asking me to hurry up, telling me she had other things to do. She seemed to think that since she spoke no English, and had no job to go to that the UK taxpayers would all just support her. My faithful interpreter was a very patient young lady, but even she was getting annoyed.

Some Home Office Immigration Officers attempt to intimidate applicants by treating them like filth. The idea is to scare them. That way they will make errors in their stories. They will reveal their true plans. I never did that; I was always polite with my customers. I didn't think I could ever do that. Right up until the moment when Mrs. Attitude sitting opposite me said: "You know it's my right to live in England with my husband." I went quiet for a couple of seconds. And then I exploded.

To hell with it all! All the things I'd wanted to say to certain customers, I said. No translator was required. I had had enough. I got to the point where I was shouting. 'If you think you have such a right to my country then take the shirt off my back as well.' I tugged off my tie and threw it at the glass barrier between us. Then I unbuttoned my shirt. I was going to throw that at her as well. But it was not like the TV. By that point, I just looked like I was stripping in front of her while yelling obscenities. I walked out of the office and slammed the door.

The Bulgarian staff looked at the demented, half dressed British Officer as he walked through the open plan office. There was only one thing I could do; go to the Consul and explain. Except I forgot to put my shirt back on. So I stood in front of her with my hairy chest displayed and my shirt dangling half on. I told her that I had made a mistake and insulted a customer. She looked at me and, without laughing, told me to get dressed, go back in, apologise, and explain that a new interview would be arranged. I did my duty, but with no enthusiasm. I stood in front of her with my hands clasped in front of me, my head down and muttered; 'I'm sorry'.

My interpreter picked up the slack by explaining that a new interview date had to be arranged with a new visa officer. I had some joy, as the woman went mental over that. The interpreter recieved flowers and chocolates later for her noble sacrifce. The application was handed over to the Immigration Officer working with us. I knew that she would face hell from the applicant after my little display. I honestly cannot recall the outcome of that, but, knowing my colleague, I doubt that Mrs. Attitude received the good news that she was after.

Chapter Nineteen: Friends

The final section in this book has to be friends, which is one of the things that you learn the most about when you end up in a situation like mine. Don't worry, no sloppy American or European rubbish will be involved here, but take it as read that I truly appreciate all of you. It's silly that you have to get a bloody disease like cancer to realise how many and what fine quality of friends that you have.

I have felt truly drawn to you all and I have really enjoyed all the visits that you have made to me, despite what I looked like early on. In many cultures there is a rite of passage that bonds members of a tribe together. The sharing of blood; joining the first hunt together or being forced to look at my testicles and penis hanging out of my pyjama trousers. We have been united in a bond that transcends all horror. No war, no blood letting, no trials or tribulations will amount to anymore than a minor inconvenience now that you have joined the Band of Bollocks. I think the one suffered the most, excluding my family of course who got the full frontal hours after the operation, must have been Mary. So well done to Mary for not being violently sick or bursting into fits of laughter. Anyone visiting me at the hospital gets to join this Masonic-like band. We should have taken photographs I guess, but my sense of humour might have been a bit extreme for the nurses.

So for those in the Band of Bollocks, I have a statement. Yes, we can support one another in all social and employment matters, but we are not having an annual reunion where I drop my trousers in the bar. If a certain Mr. Green uses his knowledge of my lower regions to any advantage other than pure and simple humour, I shall send one of my ex-wives up his trouser leg to cause him considerable pain! It is strange what a group of friends may have as a shared experience: National Service[54], Woodstock or in our case the Norfolk and Norwich hospital, my genitals and a load of mucus!

But it has been good from my point of view. Rather like a decent Christmas but without the food. I mean I've had 'Etch A Sketch'[55] (and well done, Angie as Noel will love it once Daddy has finished with it); books and puzzle books by the score. There's the famous Rod Horne cartoon which I understand hangs in the bar, will be on a wall in my house soon, and is being used as a training aid at the hospital. I also get to play board games like chess, which I love. Ok, I may be losing at the moment of writing, but I am getting healthy so beware. It may sound silly, but this bit of being ill is really

---

[54] Comupulsory service in the British Armed forces, discontinued in 1960.

[55] Popular mechanical drawing toy, first made available in 1960.

rather fun. Just don't tell the Human Resources department!

I think the only way I can thank all of you, and I mean those in Interprint, reception, retired staff, our own sweet room 101, and, of course, the Band of Bollocks, is to save up a couple of pennies and buy a round upon my safe return to my stool at the Social Club. The process may render me mute again if the prices have gone up, of course, but my expenditure is not high these days anyway. Well, it's bugger all, since I cannot eat; drink; smoke; move more than 100 yards a day; use a phone; have a shower or a bath (it's a bucket of cold water a day), and wear any clothes other than very ill-fitting pyjamas. So I think we can all have a well-deserved beer on behalf of the NHS, who have had to look after me.

One thing I have learnt is that communication without speech is a nuisance. It's hard to write fast enough, and impossible to put any emphasis on words so as to make some of my jokes work better. My parents have kept all my original scribbles for a laugh. It might be interesting to see what babbling I might have come out with over the past three-week period if I'd been able to speak. While I have been handing out messages, three people have actually written back to me, forgetting that I am mute not deaf. On the Guessing Ward, I actually have a health care worker who talks to me slowly and at increased volume as if I am some thick Frenchman. I am tempted to write a printed note in massive capital letters saying that I am unable to speak, but I can hear her fine. I do not wish to listen to your moronic babbling, but could you please continue to pick up my soiled pyjamas. She really does annoy me. All the catering staff, cleaners, other healthcare, workers, nurses, doctors, specialists, and patients treat me in exactly the same way as I was before all this happened. As a somewhat eccentric but mostly normal human being.

It goes without saying, of course, that all my friends have continued to treat me in the same way, which has been so important. My father has gone out of his way to be even more humorous with me, which is great. It is still uncertain as to what speech capability I will have in the future. Even if a little returns now, it may be lost as I go through the chemotherapy. It's the same with the ability to eat. A case of wait for another three months and see what's left of me before any more operations can be attempted. I know my friends will still love the silent movie version of me if that's the outcome.

Just to return to my friend the Almighty. The one that finds my life so amusing. He did a good thing in making me the ultimate 'Unlucky Bastard.' A chap in my old ward has skin cancer. He is the same age as me. He was a might peeved with his situation, and so was his family. There was a lot of weeping. Those kind of emotional outbursts don't really help, but my presence did. He was sat next to someone who was worse off than him. It didn't matter what problems he had day by day; my situation was always going to be worse. It ended up being funny, and he shed his last tear. He pops in to visit me from time to time now. No false sympathy, just the benefit of having an Uber 'Unlucky Bastard' assisting others by his own exceptional misfortune. It helps to be positive and enjoy whatever is happening, even if on the outside it looks bloody awful.

Now I have to stop here until I have completed the rest of the saga. As it stands, I will send it to a few friends so they can pick out bits to have a laugh at. As I said at the beginning, this is not a life story merely a collection of the disasters that have befallen me. So you are at liberty to ignore as much of it as you wish because there is no plot to follow.

Chapter 20: Memories of Mark - Reminiscences

Mark David Welsh (friend)

"I first met Mark through work, although if I were to be totally honest, it was in a bar. Specifically the bar of the Norfolk County Council Staff and Social Club, an on site establishment, completely funded and run by Council Staff.

It was lunchtime. He had a walking stick because of his hip. I had one because of my ongoing vertigo issues. Naturally we exchanged a word ot two and from there grew an unlikely lunchtime ritual; two blokes with almost nothing in common who sat together, shot the breeze, and laughed like fools. Come to think of it we did have one thing that brought us together, a shared sense of the general absurdity of life.

On more than one occasion, lunchtimes became evenings and I hold fond memories of more than a few of them. Mark injecting wine directly into his stomach with brightly coloured plastic syringes because he could no longer swallow anymore. Sitting in the kitchen of his house at 2 am on the day he was due to go into hospital for the first time, having drunk ourselves to an absolute standstill. Strange, rambling conversations when he would ring my mobile in the early hours of the morning.

So what was it about Mark? To my mind, he possessed a very rare quality. His curiosity. He was genuinely interested in people and what they had to say. He wanted to hear your opinion, your point of view, details of the things that you were passionate about. When you talked with him he wasn't sitting there working out what he would say next, waiting to interrupt you and hijack the conversation to talk about himself. He was genuinely listening to you and taking it all in. When he asked questions, it wasn't just to be polite, it was because he wanted to know the answers.

The subjects of our talks ranged from the battle tactics of great generals to the problems of a cash-strapped club in lower league football. And just about everything in between. I learnt a lot from him, and I hoped he learnt a little from me. We laughed a lot.

Editing this book was a pleasure for me because it was a little like those lunchtimes all over again. Listening to a fascinating man who had lived a full and interesting life. A man with strong opinions, some of which I do not share, but would welcome the chance to debate with him over one more pint. The fact that I cannot do that is the only regret I have about knowing Mark. Apart from the fact that he didn't include the story in his book about how he woke up drunk under the bed of a Bulgarian prostitute! Although, I suppose that was about all he could remember about it.

Save me a seat mate."

Stephen Blyth (friend)

A tribute to a friend

"He made my teenage years the Stella years and made me proud by being my Best Man at my wedding.

He will always be the best man that I had adventures with, broke bread with, prayed with and shared a passion for good rock and soul music.

Take care on your last great adventure."

Gary Green (friend)

"My friend the true English gent..........with a few quirks!

I first met Mark in a pub (probably where most people first met this wonderful man). He used to sit, not so quietly, in the corner supping on a glass of white wine, regaling people with stories of his decadent past, if you were willing to listen to them, which I was, but I can't repeat them either! Lol (lot of laughs)

Never one to shy away from a conversation, he had a gentle way about him. He spoke softly and always had a cheeky look in his eyes. No matter what life threw at him, he smiled, took a deep breath and carried on.

Even when he was diagnosed with cancer, there was no self pity (at least it didn't show), he just got on with what was left of his life by looking out for his family before worrying about himself. Even put his friends and neighbours before himself, always trying to make people feel at ease.

Then the worst happened and he passed away. He had planned to have a few mourners smiling at his funeral service; 'Always look on the bright side of life' was his choice of music and just as they carried Mark to his final resting place 'Always look on the bright side of death' was sung out. I'm not sure if that was what he had planned or whether it was Mark messing about in the 'thereafter!

I'm not ashamed to say it brought a smile to my face and I felt he was smiling back, proud that he could still get a smile from someone even after death.

Mark, I'm sure you are up there giggling away. Keep practising your chess game my friend."

Roderick Horne (colleague and friend)

"All of my early encounters with Mark were across the bar in the N.N.C. Sports and Social Club. He would usually take up station in the corner of the bar, perhaps for the support that the two sides gave him! This position is known now, to the bar staff at least, as Mark's corner.

My early encounters with him made me think he was a little odd and perhaps, sometimes, a little drunk. As I got to know him better I realised he was a little odd, but in the nicest of ways, and frequently a little drunk, but in the funniest of ways; the alcohol making some of the things he said even more outlandish. Despite me finding him a little strange in a way I can't define, I slowly warmed to the man and welcomed his sense of humour and his reminiscences during the early part of an evening shift. During this time he met and married an Albanian woman who, it appeared, he came to dislike intensely. She was soon a source of his humour, but in a bitter sort of way.

Then he developed a sore throat; this into a very harsh voice, then cancer of the throat.. I have no first hand knowledge of how people take this sort of news, but Mark was almost flippant, finding humour even in this, the worst of news. I don't think Mark was under any illusion just how serious his condition was, but his atti-

tude to such a terrible thing was but a small indication of just how bravely he would endure the absolutely awful times ahead.

Those even a little close to him watched as he dealt with his ever worsening sickness, the heartlessness of his wife and the emotional pressures of leaving his son and family, with a bravery to be admired. He would always greet his visitors with a big smile and a cheery wave no matter what sort of a day he had had.

I like to think that the three cartoons I drew, two of them inspired by comments he had made to me, for him, captured the man and his cavalier attitude to life. His bravery during those dark days and the manner, in which he faced the end, should be an inspiration to us all.

Truly, an ordinary man with an extraordinary personality."

Lindsey and Sarah (friends and work colleagues)

"We both worked in the same office as Mark although I (Lindsey) hadn't known Mark very long before he became ill. Even so, before I had even met him his sense of humour shone through from those who already knew him.

There was the legendary story of Ready Eddy, the adult superhero teddy costume (used for children's engagements). Mark brought round to my desk a large box that had been delivered to me (Sarah) Inside was a full-sized teddy bear costume that I had ordered, believe it or not, to help us promote emergency planning to children. It was to become 'Ready Eddy the Emergency Teddy'.

I insisted that Mark put the costume on so that we could check it was ok. Mark was always up for a laugh, but on this occasion he protested, as he needed to get back to his work. However I insisted and so Mark obliged and became 'Ready Eddy'. This caused lots of funny looks around the office and many laughs. However this was short lived, as a few minutes later Mark's manager came round the corner, gave him a stern look and suggested he got back to work post haste! Oops! On his return to his desk, minus the costume, Mark was scolded for his antics. I had to speak to his manager and admit it was on my insistence, that Mark had put on the costume, therefore I was to blame. I must admit he did look funny in it !

Then there was Mark's surprise birthday gathering, put on for him by his friends in the office. At this point in time, Mark was ill with cancer and was 'nil by mouth' and had a feeding tube, but he didn't let that stop him enjoying himself. He embraced the get-together with his usual enthusiasm and sense of humour. Not to mention the glass of red wine he managed to consume through his feeding tube!

My friend and I visited Mark many times at his home and kept him in touch with all that was going on at the office, as he was always interested in everyone he had worked with.

Lastly, three of us went to visit Mark in the hospice not long before he passed away and I was amazed at how he still maintained his great sense of humour. He was finding it difficult to communicate and was writing things down but joking about his bare feet poking out of the bottom of the sheet. He said he needed a pedicure and when I offered to paint his toenails for him he said he wanted them to be pink for the ladies!

This was the last time I saw Mark but I will always remember his happy nature and sense of fun.

Mick Kemp (friend)

"So, there I am. Propped up at the bar when MDW springs it on me.

Would I write something to include in a book for Mark? At first, the total blankness of sheer panic is followed by "Why me?", but then my natural arrogance comes to the fore. After all, aren't I The Man With No Brain, Fastest Punslinger in the East, always shooting From The Quip?

Surely I could come up with something. Right? Right? Wrong!

I racked my remaining brain cells in an effort to recall something about Mark that would stand out as something exceptional, unique and deeply profound.

Not a thing!

So what could I remember about him?

Well, we would usually see each other Friday after work at the club, drink some drink, and exchange the usual pleasantries.

In fact, we did what most men did when they've had a drink.

We talked some squit, put the worlds to rights, moaned about work and other people.

We weren't close friends, we never went to each other's houses, or had meals together, but we got on alright.

Then I found out that he was sick.

Like the coward that I am, I never visited him in hospital.

I suppose I prefer to remember people as hale and hearty rather than sick and dying.

Then I found out he had recovered.

I spoke to him a couple more times, but the banter was not the same.

Then I found out that he had died.

Like the coward that I am, I never went to his funeral.

So. Did I enjoy his company?

Yes!

Did he enjoy mine?

I hope so!

Do I miss him?

Hell, Yes!"

Nick Forey (Carer)

"One day I received a phone call from the office, telling me that I would be leaving where I was currently working and moving on to another package (as they were called). So I packed my bags, said my good byes and left when my replacement arrived.

The nurse practitioner, which worked for the agency, had to take me through some competencies before I went to the new client. These done, off we went to meet him.

On arrival, I was met by Mark, a short little fella wearing glasses and with a trachy (tracheotomy tube) yet a very warm, smiley little fella. After the initial meet I was shown around, sometimes you can just tell from that very first moment that you are going to get on with someone. As I was being shown around I saw pictures of Laurel and Hardy, Morecambe and Wise, Charlie Chaplin and various WWII pictures on the wall and I thought "yup, we're going to get on".

So that was it, I was left with Mark.

Without a doubt, the trip to Ypres and the WWI tour was a highlight for me but the trip was so important for Mark and his mum. Not only was it to visit the battlefields, something that Mark was hugely interested in, but it was also to visit the grave of his great uncle, who fought and died during the Great War. The journey took it out of Mark but on the first actual day of the visit we went to Hill 62. There was a memorial to the fallen Canadian soldiers on it plus it still had a partial trench system there. Mark looked so happy, to be going through the trenches, he had made it! We visited so many wonderful places with such sad histories. I have a picture of me and Mark hugging at a place called he Ulster tower, that was a good day and a good laugh with the little fella. We had such a good time, with so many happy memories.

The best memory I have of Mark is...Mark was watching a video of his son, I believe it was his son's 3rd birthday. I don't remember what I was up to but I was in the same room. The film had been on for a while when I asked Mark who it was talking on it. He said it was him, and suddenly I realised that for the first time I was hearing Mark's real voice and not the trachy affected voice I was used to. It never dawned on me that the voice I was used to, wasn't his own.

This then leads on sadly to the end. Mark's health took a sharp downwards turn once we returned from the Battlefields. His condition became harder to cope with at his house, so he went to a hospice. He still didn't lose his smile and humour; I had nothing but admiration for him. Everyone has physical strength and everyone has mental strength but Marks mental strength was huge, he kept going and going. Even when he couldn't speak he still didn't lose his sense of humour, writing everything down.

He passed away and he had the most beautiful funeral I've been to. He is buried at Colney Woods, a perfect resting place for a great friend.

There's a saying, only the good die young...I wish that wasn't the case, I miss him.

Hilary Arthur (friend and colleague from Foreign Office days)

"I first met Mark when we were working together in Sofia, where he was known to one and all as 'Tufty'. I think on account of his hair, although I never got to the bottom of that !

He'd already been there a while when I arrived and he played a huge part in helping me to settle in to a new job, and feel at home in a new country. He was welcoming and inclusive and lost no time in introducing me to his favourite haunts, his wide circle of friends and his favourite tipple –'Tranimer' white wine.

He had a great sense of humour and got on well with everyone. We soon became good friends as well as colleagues, and spent a lot of time chewing the fat and putting the world to rights in our local, 'The Boot'.

I also have great memories of trips further afield. A magical visit to Rila Monastery in the snow, a weekend in the mountains singing along to Boney M and a wonderful week in northern Thailand to celebrate our friend's wedding.

Our paths diverged when Mark left Bulgaria and we lost touch for a while, although I frequently thought about him and wondered what he was doing.

I finally got to see him again just before he passed away. Although he was pretty ill by then, he was still the same 'Tufty' I remembered from Sofia – the same upbeat spirit, the same roughish sense of humour.

He was a great guy who left a lasting 'mark' on everyone who knew him. My only regret is that we didn't manage to get back in touch sooner.

Robin Rowen (Carer)

"What can one say about Mark except he must have been one of the nicest clients I have worked for.

Even though he knew he was very ill and was nearing the end of his days, he was always so cheerful, and what a sense of humour he had. I have never laughed so much with a client as I did with him. As everyone knows he enjoyed his wine, even though he took it through his peg so had no idea of type of wine, cultivar's, flavour or taste. We used to discuss the various aspects of the wine with regard to the acids, strength, colour and taste, which he used to dream up, even though nothing was passing over his taste buds. How we joked and laughed.

With me being interested in history we had long discussions, especially on the two wars. And used to love watching the various programmes on TV together.

I also remember how excited he got when one of us were going down to London to fetch his son for the weekend. He so loved having him around and I do hope the family get to see him still.

I am so sorry I was not able to see Mark towards the end or be at his funeral but will always remember him as the three times married, Christian, Jewish and Muslim person, who had such a wonderful personality, nature and good humour that I do not think I will ever forget him."

Shirley (Trachy Nurse)

"Well, what can I say about Mark? I only knew him for a short while but we laughed, cried and laughed again. Mark was the friendliest, funniest, most comprehensive and humble person I have ever met in my life. He was always worrying about the welfare of others before himself.

Mark's favourite song was "Always see the bright side of life", and this he did regardless of the difficult situations he found himself in; trying to overcome, passing on his words of wisdom wherever he could. I can hear him saying the words of the song as I go about my job today, trying to always be as positive as him and to have a smile on my face.

My colleague and I have many good memories of Mark. Our favourite, and the one we had to chuckle over, was the day he answered his front door, not knowing it was one of us there. What's the problem you may ask? Well, he was not allowed to eat or drink by mouth due to his condition but he opened the door with a smile and a large glass of wine in one hand! The words from my colleague were " You're busted!" – but in true Mark style, with a smile and using his communication pad, he tried to convince us that he couldn't be rude. His friend had come to visit and brought a bottle of wine to share, which was very nice and how could he refuse! Ha! Ha!

Mark was a very special person and he will always be remembered."

Glenys Newton (Mark's cousin)

"Mark was my cousin but he was more than that, he was my mate.

Mark lived a full life with a big heart and it was impossible to be around him without finding yourself laughing and for the conversation to quickly tip into the ridiculous. Maybe that was the combination of the two of us as we were cut from the same cloth. Mark and I shared many of the same views on life and those that we didn't share we could talk about and both learn something new.

When Mark was ill he asked many questions about life in general and we sent long, missive emails back and forth mulling over the world in general. I treasure that. Mark may have left this earth sooner than many people but he packed several lifetimes into the 48 years that he was here and when I think of him, I always have a little chuckle. When I am doing something ridiculous, I always have a chat, as I know that he would be head in hands, but would think it was hilarious.

We both shared the view that life is an adventure to be lived, even if many a mistake is made along the way. We would have conversations around our poor life choices that had us rolling around laughing. And that's the thing about Mark, laughter. I remember him with laughter and that truly is a wonderful legacy to leave."

Karen Griffith (Mark's sister)

"I have started writing this so many times and got no further than the first sentence. How do you sum up in just a few words what someone meant to you who have been in your life as long as you have lived? Well I am sat on a train looking just staring out of the window and I can visualise Mark so clearly. I know he is around me; he is with me now. That makes it easier for me to finally do this.

Mark and I grew up like any other siblings, playing, squabbling, loads of laughs. Laughing was something I always did when Mark was around. He was just such a quirky person! He and I used to love our holidays down at the caravan in Norfolk. Crazy bike rides in the woods, precarious go-karting, flying kites on the Heath. Even simple things like sharing bunk beds and listening together to the rain dropping on the caravan roof.

Mark was a real character. His easy going relaxed nature made him great company. He had a lot of close friends and was always the life of the party. And boy did he party! From his teenage years I can remember one such time where Mark and I went on a school United Nations trip to Germany. All the countries represented there had to demonstrate their culture by way of some kind of performance. They were all serious and somewhat boring until England's performance by the very Mark Griffith! He and two friends decided to dress up in leotards and a tutu and perform an excerpt from the Nutcracker ballet! I will never forget people's faces and will always remember the roars and tears of laughter. That was the Mark we all knew. He brought a lot of fun.

As adults, we spent many years living a long way apart, particularly when Mark was working abroad. But we always knew we were there for each other. I am so grateful that Mark returned to Norwich so that we got to spend a lot of time together before he became ill.

People used to say how different Mark and I were. Well yes, looks wise we were, Mark used to always describe himself as the short, pot bellied bald one! Personality wise, yes again, quite different, but it worked. My sensible but worry head worked well with his crazy, relaxed head. We always set each other back on the right path whenever we needed it. Of course we had one big thing in common and that was sharing a bottle of wine and putting the world to rights!

Anyone who has had cancer or has cared for someone with cancer, knows just what an awful illness it is. But no matter how ill Mark felt, he never made a fuss and was always more interested in what kind of day I'd had rather than himself. He taught me what dignity in life and death was. As a close friend of his said, no matter how dark the situation, he was a true English gent with a stiff upper lip.

I know that it will be very difficult going forward without Mark in our lives. But I also know that he did not want us to be overwhelmed with sadness. He was a very strong and positive individual and would always look for the best in any situation and would want us to do the same. Let's remember Mark for all of his great qualities and appreciate the time we spent with him. Although Mark's life was cut short, we spent hours chatting during his illness and he would often say he felt he had filled his one short life with two full lives.

Of course Mark will live on in his lovely son Noel and already I can see a lot of Mark in him. Noel is a really happy soul who loves being with people, but also very much enjoys playing on his own. He loves his soldiers and has a very vivid imagination. Noel has also inherited his Daddy's great sense of fun and humour, and I know he will do well in life.

I would like to leave you with a final piece written by Mark in his last letter to me. It says "ok Karen. I'm heading back to my gang in the death lark. No doubt I have found some way to make it funny. I do not want you to be sad and that is why you must always look on the bright side of life. That is where I will be and that includes the line always look on the bright side of death because I am there too Karen. I am always smiling and trying to make your life happy for you. So if you cry too much, you will bugger up my cunning plan! I am here with you always. You know that."

Sheila Griffith (Mark's Mother)

'Never knowingly hurt anyone'

"On reading some notes Mark had made for his funeral he said 'I had a fun life but I never knowingly hurt anyone. I would like to be remembered for that.'

Mark loved life and he loved people. He found them so interesting and, in fact, thought more of others than himself. He was never bothered about material things, except as a child with his great collection of soldiers. He was never one to covert what others had but was very happy with what life presented to him. He was very much a family person and as he grew up, the one thing on his mind was to have a family of his own. He wanted to continue the life he had enjoyed as a child, with his own family. Cancer was one of the cruelest things that could have happened to him. He had his family, his dearly loved son and a home he'd always wanted and then cancer struck. His son was only two years old when Mark was told he had cancer and four when he died.

For many people this would have finished them, but Mark was made of stronger stuff. He tried not to think too far ahead but to enjoy what was around him at the time.

You will have read about his time in hospital and how he made the best of what was a very difficult illness. The hospital staff and his carers all spoke highly of him.

His son came to stay with him every other weekend and Mark cherished every moment he had with him. I would put Noel to bed and read him a story, then tell him I was going to make sure his Daddy was all right. As soon as I was downstairs I could hear Noel following me. He would then creep into the room and quietly climb up onto his Daddy's lap for a cuddle. These were Mark's favourite times with his son.

Although Mark was unable to speak or eat for most of the time he was ill, it didn't upset Noel one bit. I could see that Noel was going to grow up just like his Dad, a loving, caring person.

Mark's illness made us all, as a family, realise that we never know what life has in store for us. Take each day at a time and make the most of it. Money, although necessary for day-to-day living, is not the most important thing in life. How we behave towards each other is far more important.

Mark was a great ambassador and will be remembered for his love of people and strength of character when it mattered most. He will always be greatly missed."

Brian Griffith (Mark's Dad)

"Mark was an ordinary man with an extraordinary personality. He had the ability to immediately relate to people of all walks of life; from the children living in his street to the heads of state he met when working for the foreign office.

He started life in a small maternity hospital in Bristol and was a problem right away because the doctor was so certain that his mother had a good number of hours to go before she gave birth he decided to go home. Within 1 hour of that Mark was born with just one midwife and his father to deliver him. His time keeping has been bad ever since that first entry into the world. Many times coming home from school or work he has been hours doing a 10 minute journey putting his mother into spasms of worry and his father leaving him a note stating that his cooked meal was in the dog.

The reason for his bad timekeeping however is the indication of why he has always been so likeable. He would always be giving a helping hand to someone or listening to their problems or buying them a snack or a hot drink; completely forgetting about those at home waiting for him. Mark always put other people before himself. He would sympathise and empathise with those in trouble or sickness forgetting any problems he had himself. And he did have problems although he very rarely mentioned them or complained about them; all through his 21 months of cancer he never complained or became bitter. In fact many of the patients in hospital with him told us, his family, how much Mark had helped them and uplifted them when they were so low.

He also had epilepsy since the age of 10 and was on very strong medication to try to control it but he never let it interfere with his life nor did he impose this medical condition on his friends and family. His one big disappointment was that because of the epilepsy he could not join the army, which he so much wanted to do. But typical Mark he did not let it interfere with his living. He said in the last days of his life that although short in years he had lived a very full life and had crammed in the equivalent of two lives into his 48 years.

He will however, probably be remember mainly for his sense of humour. Whatever bad things happened to him, whatever disappointments beset him he always managed to find the funny side of them and make himself and others around him laugh. He had such a wonderful knack of seeing humour where no one else could. This with his great strength of character and determination made him a person to admire and respect. Practically everyone who met him since he was ill with cancer remarked on these wonderful traits of character. Even his solicitor who was dealing with his divorce and access to his child wrote this to us his family, and I quote " I wouldn't have thought it possible for an individual to face the prospect of death and cope with pain, with such bravery, humour and humility" Mark really was an inspiration to us all.

One last true example of his bravery and humour I leave with you. When he went into hospital for the last time the young female doctor asked him if he would sign to say he would not want to be resuscitated when his heart stopped. He looked at her and wrote down I will if you will give me a kiss. Which she did on his forehead. So he wrote down "Ah the kiss of death" and promptly signed the form. That doctor actually put that incident in Mark's medical notes much to the amusement of the senior consultant who told us about it.

Mark, we salute you. Your inspirational, brave, unselfish life will live within our hearts forever."

The Last Page: A Final Word from The Author

For some reason, at the front or the back or books you have a page that is for dedications to those that have helped in the writing of it.

Well, the main dedication is my big thanks to the bloody great cancerous growth in my head that has made all of this possible and brought together so many people by way of professional expertise, family bonds, and friendship. Naturally, we all hope that it dies a miserable death at the end of all the medical activity so that I can continue to enjoy my family and friends.

I wish to say thanks to all the people I have written about who have made me the butt of their jokes or who I have been involved with in my various disasters. A special word of thanks to Fosters Solicitors for all their assistance in clearing up my mess; particularly regarding wills, house conveyance, criminal law and family law. Especially for their repeat work on my divorces.

Naturally my thanks go to all of my wives for providing such a bedrock of humorous, bloody painful, and expensive situations.

Within the book is a list of all the roles of the medical experts involved in keeping me alive and, hopefully, curing me. This list does not even mention the catering staff, cleaners, the guys who move the beds, all variations of the nursing staff and researchers, plus three wards of dedicated professionals. Dr. Nazir and Tom are in charge of the surgical and the chemotherapy and radiology teams, but there are so many people I could mention that to start would lead to rudeness because I would miss someone out. I shall offer my thanks to you all by way of this note, and revisit this dedication at a later date and mention in despatches all those that have been dealing with me on a more daily basis.

Finally, you may have wondered why I called the book "And Now I Cannot Laugh Anymore."

Well, whatever operations I have and treatment I get, there is one thing I have definitely, and permanently, lost. The ability to laugh. I think that's rather ironic, given everything that has happened to me.

Afterword

The greatest regret Mark had was knowing he wouldn't see his son grow up, so he wrote all Noel's birthday cards up to the age of 18. He wrote suitable comments in them according to Noel's age, even telling him how to treat the girlfriends! He asked me to put a photo of himself at the same age in each card so Noel would remember his daddy as he grew up. I can't wait for Noel to see his daddy at the age of 18!

Despite his severe illness and considerable pain, Mark was an inspiration to other patients around him. He had a pair of Simpson slippers (bright yellow blobs on the ends of his legs) and every time he went into hospital he wore them. In fact, he was well known for them. Even on the way to the operating theatre, there they were sticking out from under the blanket.

The only time he didn't take them was his last visit to Priscilla Bacon Lodge, and I am sure it was because he knew he wouldn't be coming home again.

He died peacefully at 8.15pm on August 29th, 2014.

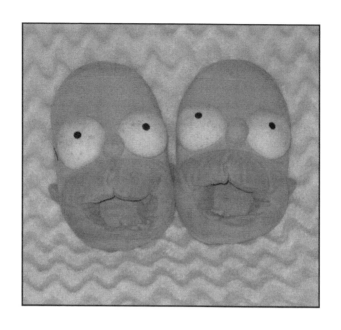

'Always look on the bright side of life…'

Monty Python

Acknowledgements

Mark's family would like to thank all those people who looked after him during his dreadful illness. The doctors, nurses and technicians at the Norfolk & Norwich Hospital, with special thanks to Dr. Tom Roques, oncologist, Mr. Ramez Nassif, ENT, Shirley and Erica, trachy nurses and Amanda, dietician. Their untiring devotion to him was amazing. Also, his GP Dr. Scouller, who allowed him to phone her anytime, day or night (even once when unknowingly she happened to be on holiday with her family). Dr. Kate Sodham and her wonderful staff at Priscilla Bacon Lodge. The ambulance teams who were so cheerful and uncomplaining as they ferried Mark back and forth to many appointments at the hospital.

The full-time carers: Rozalia, Robin, and Nick, who looked after Mark at home which such devotion and love. Their care made it possible for him to remain at home and to be with his son & and family.

Mention must be made of all Mark's work colleagues at County Hall, who visited him at home and in hospital, keeping him up-to-date on all the local gossip. Their friendship and loyalty to him made him feel normal in an abnormal world.

Peter Taylor Funeral Services for their kindness and on-going sympathy.

Marie Coe from Elizabeth Finn Care for her kindness in donating a computer to Mark, which was used to help create this book.

Finally, a very big thank you goes to his friend Mark David Welsh, who agreed to put all of Mark's ramblings together into the book he always wanted to have published. Mark David Welsh is also the author of 'Vagabond Sky', 'Kingdom of Ghosts', 'Dogs On The Highway' and others.

Profits from the sale of this book will benefit The Norfolk and Norwich University Hospital Oncology Fund. Part of the NNUH Charitable Fund (1048170)

Printed in Great Britain
by Amazon